## *Advance Praise for* HIS PROSTATE AND ME

"This is one of the most sensitive, enlightening, informative discussions of the impact of prostate cancer on a relationship I have ever read. It is written from the heart, the head and the spirit. The writing is witty, direct and serious. The information is appropriate and accurate. The insights are inspiring and, above all, hope is overflowing. Most importantly, it is a living, breathing testimony to the power of love."

*--- Dr. Andrew von Eschenbach, M.D.,*
*Director of the National Cancer Institute*
*Prostate Cancer Survivor*

"For a couple, the diagnosis of prostate cancer turns their world upside down. They are presented with bewildering and often contradictory clinical information that is difficult to assimilate and sometimes must cope with unanticipated complications of treatment, as well as the fear of tumor recurrence. All this, while the rest of the world goes on!

Desiree Lyon Howe guides couples through the emotional and clinical maze they must traverse. She offers useful advice on dealing with the stresses and depression that go with this experience. She provides accurate information about the existing treatment options and shows how, through love, faith, and understanding, their lot can be turned from tragedy to triumph."

*--- Dr. William Catalona, M.D.,*
*Professor of Urology*
*Washington University*

"This book is a must read for couples facing prostate cancer."

*--- Arnold Palmer,*
*Golfing Legend*

"This book will greatly improve the ability of families to deal with the diagnosis, treatment and side effects of this important disease."

*--- Bob Dole,*
*former U.S. Senator*

*Desiree Lyon Howe*

# HIS PROSTATE AND ME

Desiree Lyon Howe is a patient education and advocacy expert. She serves on the boards of M.D. Anderson Cancer Center and the National Organization of Rare Disorders and is the Executive Director of the American Porphyria Foundation. She lives in Houston with her husband, Dr. Richard J. Howe.

# HIS PROSTATE AND ME
## A COUPLE DEALS WITH PROSTATE CANCER

---

### DESIREE LYON HOWE

Winedale Publishing
Houston

Published by Winedale Publishing Company

Copyright © 2002 by Howewrite, Inc.

Published in the United States by Winedale Publishing Co., Houston

www.winedalebooks.com

Library of Congress Cataloging-in-Publication Data

Howe, Desiree Lyon.
His prostate and me : a couple deals with prostate cancer / by Desiree
Lyon Howe.-- 1st ed.
p. cm.
ISBN 0-9701525-7-4
1. Prostate--Cancer. I. Title.
RC280.P7 H685 2002

2002001352

Manufactured in the United States of America
2 4 6 8 9 7 5 3
First Edition

*Book Design by Babette Fraser*

To my husband, Dr. Richard Howe,
as well as to all other prostate cancer survivors
and the women who stand by their sides.

# CONTENTS

# HIS PROSTATE AND ME

# Introduction

As I mounted the podium and began my presentation on prostate cancer to the sales force of American Medical Systems, a company that manufactures devices for overcoming incontinence and impotence, I sensed that the audience was curious about how a woman could be comfortable speaking in public on such delicate subjects.

Truthfully, I wasn't entirely at ease, but I couldn't play the innocent bystander when the intimate details of my husband's treatment for side effects following prostate cancer surgery had been published in the likes of the *Reader's Digest* and *U.S. News and World Report*.

Because my husband, Dick Howe, is a noted speaker and lay authority on prostate cancer, keeping information private about the personal aspects of his diagnosis, treatment and post surgical life has been an impossible task. As I began the presentation, I felt an inward confirmation that openness was vital among prostate cancer survivors and their partners and that sharing our lives was a major part of the healing process.

In reality, I was giving this particular presentation in Dick's place. One week before his scheduled appearance, Dick had a serious accident clearing a bed of cactus at our lake home in the Texas Hill Country. As the former President of Pennzoil, Dick had been a general, of sorts, in his corporate life, but at Brooke Army Medical Center, where he was taken with four broken ribs and a punctured lung, he ranked as a lowly civilian and was promptly placed in a ward with other men.

There we were, four men peacefully sleeping in their hospital beds behind privacy curtains and me unsuccessfully attempting to sleep next to Dick in a cumbersome, lumpy chair. I was already awake when the usual clamor started in the ward at 5 AM, the morning after our midnight arrival. I quickly roused from my chair and headed to the restroom to freshen up for the day.

When I returned to the ward at 5:15, I heard Dick lecturing the other bedridden patients about prostate cancer, the PSA test, treatments, side effects and exciting new research advances. I groaned at the thought of having to listen to this before my morning coffee, and I felt sorry for the other patients who could not escape Dick's sunrise monologue. However, as the men eagerly posed a number of familiar questions and I heard Dick answer them with educated ease, I understood once again that Dick's "ministry" was for any time and any place. I understood further that, as the wife of a prostate cancer survivor, I had a major role in this calling. My support was emotionally important to him, as was my willingness to provide everything from a listening ear to assistance with the development of his next prostate cancer presentation.

Standing in for Dick at the sales meeting wasn't the kind of activity I had envisioned embarking on when we met. My closest friend, Joanne Davis, introduced Dick and me over a lovely dinner at a quaint French restaurant in busy, booming Houston. Unbeknownst to Joanne, one of her other guests decided to bring a radio sex therapist as his dinner partner. Despite the fact that anything I had to say was deadly dull compared to the sex therapist's subject matter, Dick and I shared intermittent bits of compatible conversation. Over dessert, we discovered that we had a more than average interest in medicine, a circumstance that provided Dick with the perfect opening to enlighten me on his diagnosis of prostate cancer and subsequent surgery.

Within a week after our introduction, Dick mentioned that he had suffered some side effects from the surgery, in particular moderate incontinence and impotence. Within a month, he explained the steps he had taken to deal with some of these side effects and commented that he was still trying to find good solutions to his problems. Discussing such subjects somehow didn't bother me, because it fit with my already frank nature. Another reason was that my deceased husband,

James Lyon, died after a lengthy struggle with pancreatic cancer, and I was accustomed to cancer related discussions.

When we met, Dick and I were both widowed and wandering around in what he describes as the "fog of grief" after our mates died. Both of us had been very much in love with our spouses and were devastated at their deaths. Our common interest in medicine gave us an absorbing field upon which to center our thoughts and a gratifying purpose for the future to help ease the painful agony of the losses we had sustained. Dick and I enjoyed working together, writing together, being together and recovering together from the greatest blow of our lives. Over time, our fondness grew into more than just companionship.

Cancer was not the culprit that almost ended our budding romance. That occurred one evening when Dick invited me to his home for dinner and a "really exciting video," that he hadn't yet had the opportunity to watch. When I arrived at his house, I discovered that dinner was to be whatever I could scrape together from his basically empty refrigerator. I micro-waved bits and pieces of his unappetizing leftovers, tossed them onto a TV tray and settled in front of the television for a good movie. Dick slid in the video while I started eating.

On the screen appeared the title of the film, *A Radical Prostatectomy*. I watched in horror as Dr. David Crawford, a famous surgeon, began the operation. Although the surgeon was demonstrating the latest nerve and blood sparing techniques, it was still too much for me. I quietly finagled the keys out of my purse and decided to give Dick an excuse for my early departure. But when I caught sight of the sincere, boyish interest on his face as he watched each incision, my annoyance eased. Because his educational undertaking was not selfishly motivated, I was more forgiving of this less than romantic dinner date than I would have been had his motives been totally self indulgent. Mostly, I reasoned, "This man knows absolutely nothing about courting a woman!" Such ignorance coupled with his altruistic nature were reasons enough for me to forgive him, sneak my car keys back into my purse, and pick up a magazine just as the whole prostate was being lifted from the patient's pelvic cavity.

In one way, the video experience was good for me. It made clear that if I chose to go forward with Dick, openness about his condition and taking advantage of worthy educational opportunities would be his *modus operandi*.

His desire for learning about prostate cancer eventually became mine as well, and I know that many partners, mothers, daughters, granddaughters, nieces, daughters-in-law or friends of men diagnosed with prostate cancer have the same quest.

It is my hope that this book will provide these women with practical information about prostate cancer and insight into the role they can play to help the men they love deal with this crisis. Perhaps, sharing some of Dick's and my own journey may help, as well.

# 1.

## Support

Our courtship continued in an equally unusual manner. Along with dinners on the town, we attended prostate cancer related conferences, lectures at M.D. Anderson Cancer Center and support group meetings, including many that featured Dick as the speaker.

Support groups offer excellent opportunities for prostate cancer survivors and their partners to hear good presentations about prostate cancer and to meet other survivors who are generally eager to share helpful information gained from personal experience.

I mention support groups early in this book because communicating with other couples helps reduce the emotional pressure the patient and his partner feel after a cancer diagnosis. These groups provide invaluable sources of information and encouragement during the initial period when anxiety levels are high, as well as long after treatment when the disease is cured or held at bay. Research has repeatedly shown that this kind of emotional support diminishes the fears and stresses associated with a cancer diagnosis.

Finding a group is usually easy. There are a number of prostate cancer support groups from which to choose in medium to large cities, and generally, there is at least one group in small towns. National organizations include US TOO! International and Man To Man, and there are many citywide independent gatherings, as well.

By and large, information about these support networks is listed in the local media, on the Internet or on the notice board in the urologist's office. (For a list of resources and contact information, please see Appendices, beginning on page 164.)

Although the presentations at these groups are superb and extremely beneficial, coffee time before the meeting is one of the most productive half-hours of a couple's post diagnosis life. At the refreshment tables, persons attending the meeting exchange hope and helpful tips, ranging from recommendations about good books on prostate cancer and comparisons of PSA's to guidance about a great local restaurant and news about the latest treatment developments.

These monthly gatherings are generally open to patients and their families. Some groups assemble for educational presentations or discussions simultaneously with the women attendees. Others meet separately or have time set aside in order to provide the partners with a same sex environment in which to discuss sensitive subjects like sexual problems and incontinence. These same sex meetings also provide information on an array of skills that are useful for coping with the emotional upheaval that these side effects can precipitate.

As a whole, most of the survivors in these groups represent a wide range of treatment choices and are willing to discuss their specific treatments objectively and in detail. These group members are the front line troops supporting the great assemblage of prostate cancer survivors in the United States, who now rank 1.5 million men strong.

One veteran of the support group brotherhood is Rex Zeiger, who has greatly benefited from involvement in an US TOO support group in the Scottsdale area. After his diagnosis and treatment for prostate cancer, he encountered an unexpected and unwelcome side effect of his disease: Depression. Fortunately, his wife, Ann, noticed a small advertisement that provided the toll free telephone number for the national office of the US TOO prostate cancer support group. She phoned the organization's Chicago headquarters and was given the location of a small local meeting in the Scottsdale, Arizona area.

It is interesting to note that most initial calls to the US TOO hot line are from women, like Ann. At her behest, Rex agreed to attend the meeting where he not only encountered a great group of prostate cancer survivors but also discovered a new, meaningful purpose for his life. He joined the group and later became the US TOO regional director for Arizona, where, under his leadership, there are now thirteen thriving support groups. Ann is by his side in these endeavors, and together she and Rex have made a tremendous impact in the lives of many other prostate cancer survivors.

Although Rex had found his encounter with depression surprising, it is not unusual to be overwhelmed, heavy hearted or depressed after a cancer diagnosis. The gloomy portrayal of cancer survival in years past still darkly shades the hopes of many people who are ill informed about amazing new advances in cancer treatment and the greatly improved survival rates. There have never been as many dedicated people working on a cure for cancer. There have never been as many promising treatments and strategies to overcome the disease, and there have never been as many people undergoing these treatments and living happy healthy lives because of them. Even chemotherapies are now more effective with fewer side effects than in the past.

The encouraging reality is that, if prostate cancer is caught early, men can usually achieve a cure for the disease. Unfortunately, however, men often miss early diagnosis because they tend to ignore or deny their basic health needs. Principally these involve an annual physical, which includes a digital rectal examination (DRE) and a PSA test, starting at age fifty or earlier for men at high risk, like those who have prostate cancer in the family or are African-American.

The level of denial is striking. Although a recent national survey of 1500 men over thirty-five years old recognized that prostate cancer is as serious a threat for them as breast cancer is for women, only 19% of those who were not already diagnosed with prostate cancer had discussed the probability of contracting it with their physician. Two thirds of this group identified the disease as a leading cause of death among men, but 58% of them reported that they thought it was not likely that they would be diagnosed with the disease. This degree of resistance should show women that, if they didn't know it already, their man needs help!

In fact, many women have pressed the men in their families into taking their first PSA test, thus saving their lives with early detection.

Although it's not uncommon for men to maintain silence about any illness they might contract, the idea of prostate cancer triggers the additional, almost paralyzing, fear of incontinence--the inability to control urination--and impotence--the inability to achieve a satisfactory erection. (Instead of impotence, most medical professionals use the more accurate phrase erectile dysfunction (ED).) Having, or fearing, either problem can make men less likely to communicate about their disease and less likely to investigate solutions promptly.

Dick's openness about his disease has greatly facilitated our ability to deal with its after effects in daily life, as well as allowing him to provide helpful information to large numbers of other people. It is important, however, to remember that some men choose to be silent, not because they are embarrassed about the disease, but because they are fearful of the effect their diagnosis can have on their careers.

I became aware of this one evening during a small dinner party at our home. Several of the men attending were prostate cancer survivors, including one gentleman who was well-known in the media industry. He was very "hush-hush" about his condition, even though there had been mention of it in the national news. Another of the guests, who was also a prostate cancer survivor, had heard about the other guest's diagnosis and in his usual friendly manner, approached the gentleman and merely mentioned that he too had prostate cancer. It was not done in a manner to invade his privacy but rather as a welcoming gesture, an attempt to find a common subject of conversation. Sadly, the man quickly rebuffed our affable friend. I later discovered that he and his wife were afraid such discussions would hurt his public image. In their view, once the cancer was treated that was the end of the problem and also the end of any need for discussing it.

Dick and I learned a great deal during that interchange. Mainly, we were reminded to tread lightly until a man or woman is ready to communicate about health problems, cancer or otherwise. Next, we saw again that although denial can be dangerous, it is not our place to change this disposition. It is only our place to cultivate openness by being ready to share our own experiences when the opportunity arises.

There are many well-known couples, in fact, who are sharing their prostate cancer experiences in valuable and highly public venues.

One of these is Herbie Mann, the legendary jazz flutist, and his lovely wife, Janeal. Dick and I learned about their involvement several years ago at the annual CaPCURE scientific retreat at Lake Tahoe. The goal of CaPCURE, founded in 1993 by Michael Milken after his own diagnosis, is to support prostate cancer research that will rapidly translate into treatments and cures. The annual retreat gives scientists the opportunity to share their research with one another in a beautiful setting--although the word "retreat" may be a misnomer as the participants attend meetings from dawn to late in the evening. To date, CaPCURE has contributed more than $70 million to prostate cancer research and awareness programs.

This forum presented Herbie with the perfect opportunity to enlighten participants on the vision he and Janeal share of improving public awareness about prostate cancer, with a particular emphasis on encouraging men to take the PSA test.

Herbie told his story in his easy manner to many of the participants, including Dick and me. Janeal was equally communicative about their situation and had the same comfortable, warm personality. When I met them, I thought that these two were going to be a powerful team, and they have proven that to be true.

Herbie's experience began with erectile dysfunction resulting from decreased testosterone levels. When his doctor placed him on regular testosterone injections, his condition--and life in general--improved, until Janeal's brother, a V.A. Hospital nurse, asked Herbie about his PSA.

Herbie had never heard of the PSA, but he took note and requested that his doctor give him the test. When the PSA result came back, it was a double-digit number. (For a discussion of the PSA test, see pages 41-2.) His subsequent positive biopsy was accompanied by the shocking news that his prostate cancer was inoperable. He and Janeal were devastated. However, they decided to turn their experience into a positive force by helping other men and women know that they are not alone in their dealings with this illness.

They began their mission in the midst of Herbie's treatment which first involved radiation therapy that, unfortunately, did not work for long. Thereafter, he began an experimental trial with an aggressive chemotherapy being tested at M.D. Anderson Cancer Center in Houston, which halted the cancer.

His next step was to find a way to use his talent to motivate men to get their PSA tests and, in turn, play a role in saving them from the bleak predicament he and Janeal had been facing. He began by delivering his message at concerts and other media events through a short personal testimony.

As part of this ongoing awareness campaign, Herbie has held a series of concerts around the country where the attendees were given free PSA tests on site.

The first of these "Pied Piper" concerts, held in Houston early in 2001, was a huge success. Of the 1200 attendees, 500 men were tested and each one was given a free Herbie Mann CD for their participation.

As part of their publicity campaign for the concert, Herbie and Janeal were guests on a popular daytime television show. After describing their commitment to promote prostate cancer awareness, they told the audience about a greater commitment--the one they had to each other. They explained that they treasure their relationship and spend peaceful, quiet time together early each morning as a way of fostering their oneness. Their devotion was evident to all the viewers who watched their interaction.

Herbie performs about thirty concerts around the country each year and sets aside a portion of the proceeds for the Herbie Mann Prostate Cancer Awareness Music Foundation, which is used to underwrite his free concerts and free prostate cancer-screening program.

New York Yankees manager Joe Torre and his wife Ali have also joined the prostate cancer awareness bandwagon. "I was numb when I got the diagnosis, so I don't know what I would have done without Ali," Torre says. "She sought out information, asked questions and helped guide us through the complicated process of reaching a treatment decision."

The Torres have helped launch a mentoring program called "Two Against One: Couples Battling Prostate Cancer." The goal of this program is to help communicate over the Internet with other families who have faced the challenge of prostate cancer.

Arnold Palmer, the famous golfer, has been another exceptional advocate for prostate cancer awareness. Recently, he starred in an excellent Pennzoil television commercial encouraging men to have their PSA tests. Additional information about PSA testing and prostate cancer was contained in a brochure featuring Arnold, which was distributed nationally through Jiffy Lube oil change centers. Thousands of men responded to this effective program.

Arnold has also been involved in other public awareness and research funding activities for all types of cancer, a worthy example of one man reaching out to make a difference in the lives of his fellow cancer survivors.

A few other notable survivors who have spoken out to enhance prostate cancer awareness include: General Norman Schwartzkopf, Charlton Heston, Jerry Lewis, Robert Goulet, Jesse Helms, Hamilton Jordan, Michael Korda, Andy Grove, Bishop Desmond Tutu, Richard Petty, Harry Belafonte, Stan Musial, Len Dawson, Justice Paul Stevens, Robert Novak, Mayor Rudy Giuliani, and Nelson Mandela.

The most visible prostate cancer survivor is Senator Bob Dole who was treated for prostate cancer in 1992 with a radical prostatectomy. Since then he has enthusiastically enhanced prostate cancer awareness through a number of national media campaigns, even openly discussing his use of Viagra, the drug used to treat E.D. What also interested me was his admission in a *People* magazine article that when he felt "stunned, pressured, or plain old sick," he sought help from his wife, Elizabeth, who was then head of the American Red Cross. She accessed information and physicians for him and gave him the kind of reassurance and comfort that he most needed.

Plenty of men have told me that when they, too, are "stunned, pressured or plain old sick," they quickly turn to their wives or partners for comfort. I find this same reaction with Dick. Although he encountered significant stresses as the president of a major corporation and was, therefore, accustomed to dealing with problems of great magnitude, he is sometimes fretful over small pressures. He handles them well as long as I maintain a loving, patient attitude that gives him the reassurance he needs. Even one small understanding gesture can turn the tide of a stressful circumstance in Dick's life.

Not only do men need an added measure of attention during the trying times that occur after a cancer diagnosis, but it is also not unusual for men to hand over the day-to day management of their cancer to the woman in their life. As this suggests, a woman's reactions and subsequent actions after her partner is diagnosed are vitally important in the healing process and in fostering the healing partnership.

Florence Baskas is a prime example of a loving wife who managed her husband's care with the nursing instinct of Florence Nightingale and the business acumen of the CEO of General Motors.

When her husband Morris was diagnosed with prostate cancer the disease was very aggressive. Florence immediately leapt into the fray. She became a remarkable one-woman battalion who understood the critical role of a caregiver and was ready to undertake any task that would help Morris. She bought books on the subject of prostate cancer, searched the Internet to broaden her knowledge, tracked down experts on the disease, and she called Dick and others multiple times with her long and growing list of technical questions.

After overhearing many of the conversations between Dick and Florence, I pictured Florence at her kitchen table command post poring over copious medical notes before she presented the most important facts to Morris for his review and input. It was evident that her unwavering love for Morris infused her with the strength to meet the challenges ahead instead of being overwhelmed by them.

Florence is a born giver so, when she discovered that there was not a prostate cancer support group in her area, she contacted Terry Roe, the New Jersey based regional director of US TOO, who helped her form a successful group near her home in Broxville, New York. She wanted other men and women to benefit from the knowledge, experience and encouragement couples could provide in such venues. This same group later played an important role in supporting Florence after Morris died.

As a means of both honoring Morris' life and coping with the devastating grief she felt following his death, Florence has continued her crusade to combat prostate cancer, including her work with support groups. She is a wonderful, involved wife whose example is a call to action for us to use whatever gifts we have been given to become intrinsically involved as lifelines for the men we love

There is no limit to the importance of a woman's role in combating her partner's illness. Florence chose to start a support group, but there are countless other ways in which a woman can make her own impact on the fight against prostate cancer.

Her first major influence can be on the physical and emotional health of her husband after his diagnosis. Here attitude counts. I remember once walking into the hospital room of a man undergoing treatment for prostate cancer who was very active in support groups and well educated about his condition. I had been heading out the door to visit another patient at that particular hospital, when Dick asked me to stop by this man's room and visit him as well. I had only met the gentleman a few times, so I was confused when he seemed overly glad to have my company. It didn't take long to understand why.

During our short visit, his wife continually complained about the long days and the confinement she felt when visiting her husband in the hospital. I couldn't believe it when she whined about the lack of certain television channels and the length of the walk from the parking lot to her husband's hospital room. After a few minutes of listening to her incessant carping, I wondered how this man could ever have any incentive to get well.

A few days afterwards, Dick and I visited another gentleman undergoing surgery for prostate cancer. His wife, who was staying with him in the hospital, had placed cheerful notes and photos from family and friends on every spot of usable space and had single-handedly made his hospital room a happy place. Plus, she maintained such an uplifting attitude that Dick and I commented on how fortunate her husband was to be enveloped in such a wonderful loving and healing atmosphere. We also discovered that his wife, eager to learn practical information about her husband's disease, was in the process of locating a support group network in their area for when they returned home.

# 2.

## The New Men in Your Life

Before I begin to explain the basics of the diagnosis and treatment of prostate cancer, I want to introduce you to a few of the men and women who have made the improved survival rates of prostate cancer possible.

Meeting these extraordinary men and women and observing their commitment gave me the assurance that Dick and all other prostate cancer survivors are in caring, gifted hands. I mention these doctors and their other outstanding colleagues, because they hold immeasurable sway over our lives. Their work has vastly improved the diagnosis and treatment for prostate cancer and eventually will provide the basis for a cure for the men in our lives.

One outstanding prostate cancer specialist is Dr. Andrew von Eschenbach, who was Chairman of the Department of Urology at M.D. Anderson Cancer Center at the time of our introduction. Dr. von Eschenbach is as famous for his loving personality as he is for his outstanding accomplishments and expertise. "Dr. Von," as he is fondly called among the hospital staff, should star in a documentary about doctor/patient relationships because of his extraordinary ability to educate, treat and comfort prostate cancer patients, all at the same time. One survivor recently told me that when he is discussing his case with "Dr. Von," the good doctor is so attentive that he feels as if he is his only patient.

If your partner has already had treatment, you know the significance of a good doctor/patient relationship and the negative consequences of a bad one. Although these interpersonal skills are important, they have less significance if the doctor's medical or surgical skills are not outstanding. In Dr. von Eschenbach's case, he is endowed with both, a perfect combination.

Dick was very fortunate in that his involvement on a number of national prostate cancer committees kept him in frequent contact with Dr. von Eschenbach and a friendship developed between them. Eventually, we also met his wife, Madelyn, who displays an equally dynamic personality and fervent commitment to helping secure a victory over cancer. In fact, Dr. von Eschenbach has gone on to become the President-Elect of the American Cancer Society and shortly thereafter, gave up that position to become the Director of the National Cancer Institute, the largest cancer research institute in the world.

Among the other noted men and women in the field is Dr. Patrick Walsh, Chairman of the Department of Urology at Johns Hopkins in Baltimore, Maryland. Dr. Walsh is credited with developing both the blood sparing and nerve sparing techniques used to reduce or eliminate the need for transfusion and to decrease impotence and incontinence, respectively. I eagerly anticipate every conference, which features Dr. Walsh on the program. What awaits Dick and me, if time permits, is not only a brilliant presentation by Dr. Walsh but a private dinner with him afterwards, where we are privy to his personal views on the latest prostate cancer developments and his hobby, telling great jokes. Like so many other cancer specialists, he is devoted to his patients and is intent on finding a cure for prostate cancer.

We were also fortunate to add Dr. Peter Scardino, another celebrated physician, to our extended circle of friends in the prostate cancer arena. He is a charismatic surgeon, who has impacted the world of prostate cancer with his extraordinary surgical abilities and his significant research achievements. As a testimony to his surgical expertise, men fly from points around the globe to have him perform their surgery. Dr. Scardino is not only a preeminent surgeon who has developed surgical techniques that help to preserve normal bladder and sexual function, but he is also an expert in early detection and a pioneer in gene therapy.

Several years ago, Dr. Scardino left Baylor College of Medicine in Houston to serve as the Chairman of the Department of Urology at Memorial Sloan-Kettering Hospital in New York City. The East Coast received an immeasurable blessing and Houston lost a substantial asset when this great surgeon and scientist moved to New York. Fortuitously, Dr. Scardino and Dick are still members of several important committees together, so their relationship and mutual respect has continued in spite of the distance gap.

In the course of my attendance at prostate cancer conferences, I also met many other "greats" in the field, including Dr. William Catalona from St. Louis. His very steady, humble presence earned my immediate respect. Dick's life was saved directly through Dr. Catalona's retrospective study of the PSA test, which already existed but was only FDA approved to monitor men who had been treated for prostate cancer. Dr. Catalona's study, which involved 5000 men, determined that this simple PSA test was effective for detecting prostate cancer at an early stage.

Fortunately, Dick was listening to the radio one morning in 1991 and heard about Dr. Catalona's research. As a result of this radio spot, Dick asked his internist to order it, which proved to be the life saving step that led to his early prostate cancer diagnosis. (For a full discussion of the PSA test, see pages 41-2.)

Because this simple blood test saved his life, Dick has personally thanked Dr. Catalona many times for the part he played in the process.

Then there is Dr. Donald Coffey, who belongs in a class of his own. He is a very big man with an even bigger, jovial personality and passion for life. His intellect and perspicacity are so astounding that many of us have jokingly speculated that he is some super intelligent alien life form instead of a "good guy" from Tennessee. Dr. Coffey holds five professorships at Johns Hopkins medical institutions in urology, oncology, pathology, pharmacology, and electron sciences, which is an extraordinary accomplishment, especially when most of his expertise was gained outside the classroom.

For laypersons, Dr. Coffey's special talent is his ability to present even the most technical of medical topics in an understandable manner. Plus, he teaches with such enormous enthusiasm and hope that his zeal for the subject is contagious.

Aside from his numerous scientific accomplishments, Dr. Coffey is admired for encouraging young physicians and scientists, spurring them on with his own sense of curiosity, compassion and determination to make this a cancer-free world. We are indeed fortunate that he has been involved in prostate cancer research for twenty-five years.

Many men with advanced prostate cancer are patients of Dr. Christopher Logothetis, who is the Chairman of the Department of Genitourinary Medical Oncology at M.D. Anderson Cancer Center. Most people agree that it is hard to find words to describe this compassionate, gentle genius. As an oncologist/researcher, he has the responsibility of treating men whose primary treatments have failed. His is an extremely complex undertaking that he performs with loving devotion to each of his patients and has made substantial progress in the field of chemotherapy and other treatments on their behalf.

Another important name in the world of prostate cancer is Dr. Otis Brawley, Director of the Office of Special Populations Research at the National Cancer Institute, a division of the National Institutes of Health, our nation's largest research center. Part of the focus of Dr. Brawley's work is to raise the standard of health care for his fellow African-American men. This is quite an undertaking since African-Americans have the highest incidence of and death rate from prostate cancer in the United States. Some recent reports indicate that the mortality rate of African Americans has declined from cancer in general, due in part I am sure, to the dedication of Dr. Brawley.

Dr. Norman Greenberg, a professor of molecular and cellular biology and urology at Baylor College of Medicine, plays a different but equally important role in the field of prostate cancer. We call Dr. Greenberg the "mouse man," because his research involves building genetically engineered mouse models in which the cells are preprogrammed to spontaneously develop cancer. Mouse models are frequently used to help scientists understand how different cancers develop and how they respond to different outside influences and treatments. Dr. Greenberg's mouse models allow researchers to test over a short span of time whether specific drugs or gene therapies can prevent tumor development.

This noted researcher has developed a revolutionary mouse model for prostate cancer, the autochthonous transgenic adenocarcinoma of the mouse prostate, better known as the TRAMP nude mouse model. Because these "nude mice" are born without an immune system, they are receptive to disease. Transgenic means that they can be infected with cancer, namely prostate cancer, which behaves similarly to prostate cancer in humans. His mouse model differs from traditional models in that these models are based on the injection of pre-existing tumor cell lines. I wanted to design underwear for his nude mice but tossed the idea when I discovered that there were almost a million mice living in his "mouse house."

Radiation treatment also has its leading exponents. At one time, a prostate cancer tumor was considered radiation resistant. Dr. Malcolm Bagshaw and his colleagues at Stanford University demonstrated that high-dose, small-field radiation could allow selected patients to undergo potentially curative radiation therapy instead of surgery. This pioneering work was particularly important for patients who could not endure surgery because of other medical difficulties or personal preferences against surgery.

Dr. Bagshaw also developed techniques to shield the rectum, anal canal and sphincter, pubic bone, small bowel and portions of the urethra from radiation. Considering Dr. Bagshaw's first major study on the role of radiotherapy in prostate cancer was published in 1965, his contribution is profound. Dick was honored to serve with him on the Prostate Health Council for three years.

Women, like Dr. Leslie Schover, have also changed the world of prostate cancer. Dr. Schover, associate professor of behavioral science at MD Anderson Cancer Center, focuses her research on problems that men and women experience after genitourinary and gynecologic cancer treatment.

She has published many of her findings about sexuality and cancer, which have been helpful to many couples needing to enhance their sexual relationship after one of them has had cancer treatment. She has a frank, tell-it-like-it-is approach, which is rare in the sexual arena.

All of us have our own list of medical heroes. I have only mentioned a few of the physicians and researchers whose extraordinary abilities in the fields of oncology, surgery, research, radiation, etc. have directly impacted our lives. If space allowed, I would name and individually praise every man and woman who work so diligently for the million plus prostate cancer survivors alive today. If they are not already familiar to you, many of these individuals will become familiar, because of the part they play in enhancing and sustaining the lives of your loved ones. Over time, you will add many more heroes to your own list, and they will not all be medical professionals. You, your partner and the many other amazing people who will encourage and support you will be on the list, as well. The relationship between the

21

medical team, the partners and the "encouragers" is vital to successful treatments and medical care.

## 3.

### Educating Myself

With the example of these physicians and researchers as our champions, Dick and I decided that we needed to educate ourselves on the basic principles about human anatomy, biology and physiology, so we attended a mini-medical school held for laymen at the Baylor College of Medicine in the Texas Medical Center. This was a special course devised for people in the Houston community who wanted to gain a better understanding of general anatomy and physiology and how they apply to medicine. The course taught us everything from the basics of how the heart works to how cells divide, all of which has helped us better understand the broad principals of cancer and cancer treatment. It also enabled us to add a great number of words to our limited medical vocabulary.

You may find that your community offers a similar course, but if not, you might suggest that it would be a good undertaking for your own community hospital. The attendance was exceptionally good at ours and would, I am sure, be equally so everywhere, especially since people are becoming more involved in their own medical care.

Sporting my mini-medical school diploma, I felt compelled to live up to my graduation vows to continue my education by diving into Dick's treasure trove of books and technical papers on prostate cancer.

Since most of the technical articles from prestigious medical journals, like *The Journal of Urology* and *Urology* were way over my head, I depended on books for my basic prostate cancer education. I especially liked Bill Martin's book, *My Prostate and Me*. Dick and I have recommended it to many of our men and women friends, whether they had prostate cancer or not, because it was so moving, humorous and informative. Throughout his book, Bill, who is an accomplished author and Professor of Sociology at Rice University in Houston, gives the reader not just a peek, but an open window into his heart, his family life and his personal experience with prostate cancer. I laughed and cried through each chapter and when I finished it, I found that I had received an invaluable basic education on prostate cancer in the process. We are eagerly awaiting the second edition. Bill's book spurred my thirst to read more, so I consumed many other excellent texts from Dick's sizable library.

Dr Patrick Walsh has written two extremely comprehensive books on prostate cancer, *The Prostate: A Guide for Men and the Women Who Love Them* and *Dr Patrick Walsh's Guide To Surviving Prostate Cancer*, which is an outstanding A-Z handbook that addresses issues from pre-diagnosis to long after treatment. I was happy also to see his superb glossary at the end of the book. Usually, when I come upon a medical term I don't understand, I drag out the heavy medical dictionary and plow through it until I find the term. Most often, I find that the explanation is filled with more words I am forced to look up. His book, however, is easy to read and if there is a medical term that needs defining, the glossary is easily understandable as well.

I also scrutinized many of the 400,000 prostate cancer web sites on the Internet but soon was overwhelmed by the sheer number. The more educated I became, however, the more able I was to detect blatant misinformation in the less than reliable sites. Thus I concentrated on those designed by noted institutions.

Although these websites were informative, I retained more of what I was reading when I had a real book in front of me and a yellow marker in my hand to underline the central points. Old habits die very hard.

It is interesting to note, here, that the plethora of books, journal articles, television specials and related news articles that I was enjoying were a far cry from the void Dick found on his initial search for information ten years ago. At that time, there were no books on prostate cancer for lay consumption, no brochures, no Internet and just a few newly formed support groups.

(Details on great reading matter and other resources are given in the Appendices, beginning on page 164.)

# 4.

## Our New Agendas—Dietary and Lifestyle Issues

In fact, I didn't mind such forays into the world of medicine. Through my own experience with a genetic disease called acute intermittent porphyria, a painful, life-threatening illness, I had already learned this important lesson: People who actively seek education about their own illness generally fare better than those who quietly sit on the sidelines.

What I did mind was foregoing a social life outside of the prostate cancer world. Dick had become so absorbed in his quest for knowledge about prostate cancer and his involvement in the many related responsibilities and activities that the rest of his life followed a stringent course with few social interruptions. In other words, the disease "ruled the roost."

In time, that situation grated on me, so I decided to work incrementally toward creating a more balanced life for us than Dick's work-all-day and work-all-night routine with sporadic interruptions to watch "The Sopranos" and "Wheel of Fortune." I am not so sure we came to a compromise; rather I think, after first acquiring a more than hefty dose of prostate cancer education, I just usurped his social schedule and placed myself in charge. I began planning dinners with friends and organizing exciting trips, in the conviction that this more balanced approach to life was healthier for both of us.

Although Dick adapted to the novel social agenda I organized for him, he didn't appreciate my maneuvers to change his life by placing him on a different diet regimen. Having delved into plenty of cancer prevention books, I was convinced that a diet heavy in fats was definitely not a healthy food choice. I tried to exchange Dick's favorites like steak, cheese and sausage for the likes of broccoli, assorted greens and squash. He didn't outwardly revolt. He just scooted his food around his plate and ate very little of it. Next, he started stopping at Otto's Bar-B-Q near our home in Houston, the James Coney Island Hot Dog joint or some other yummy spot for lunch and would then skittishly inform me that he was too stuffed to eat dinner. I knew then that I was losing the food exchange battle.

But I made big strides in the diet war via another unexpected tactic, not of my own devising. One of our friends is Dr. Michel DeBakey, the world famous heart surgeon. Despite the fact that he is in his nineties, Dr. DeBakey maintains a rigorous travel and work schedule. One evening, when we were hosting a dinner party at our home, Dr. DeBakey and his beautiful wife, Katrin, arrived a few minutes late, because Dr. DeBakey had just returned to Houston from Russia where he had been overseeing the surgery and care of the then Russian President, Boris Yeltsin. Dick and I were astounded that Dr. DeBakey appeared so vigorous after an intercontinental flight, especially since we are exhausted after cross-country travel and in a state of near collapse after international flights. I boldly asked him how he could maintain his strenuous daily schedule and remain so energetic after such a lengthy journey.

First, he attributed his happiness and vitality to Katrin, who is an extraordinary woman. He added that his healthy lifestyle was also important. His remark provided me with the perfect opportunity to ask Dr. DeBakey about his diet in hopes that some of his answers would rub off on Dick.

I thought Dr. DeBakey would enumerate a complicated formula of low fat, high fiber foods, but I was surprised when his response was simply that he ate a wide variety of foods, including what I call the "f" word—fat—but always only one third of what was on his plate. Furthermore, he walked miles each day during the course of his work at the Methodist Hospital, his workplace for half a century. As an aside, Dr. DeBakey added that in his seventy years as a practicing physician, he could state that people of faith and people who have purposeful lives live longer than individuals with no faith and few future goals.

Speaking with Dr. DeBakey and observing the astonishing results of his own eating and walking habits accomplished what I had tried to do for months. Dick quickly adopted the DeBakey plan. He had already begun a walking regime with me, but he now added more enthusiasm to his exercise program and began eating only a third of the food on his plate, at least part of the time.

Katrin played an equally important role in our lives. Whereas Dr. DeBakey physically repairs hearts, Katrin spiritually enlarges them. Recently, she called to invite us to dinner and at the end of our conversation, she added, "The theme of our dinner Saturday night is 'Life in the Fullest'." These are not just words with Katrin but her essence.

She envelopes her friends with love in astoundingly creative ways. Her dinner tables are decorated with original creations of natural fruits, vegetables, leaves, and herbs of all kinds, mostly grown in her lush garden. Plus, her food is always a fresh, delicious, colorful feast for the eyes more unique and imaginative than any you have seen featured in magazines. The overall experience is cozy yet overflowing with stimulating conversation. What better way to hold cancer at bay than to saturate our immune systems with pleasant times and a general state of happiness?

Prior to adopting our new DeBakey eating habits, I called Dick the "paper boy," because he spent most of his waking hours reading, writing, shuffling, copying, printing, filing and even shredding papers, none of which constitutes an aerobic activity. However, the paperwork did fulfill the last part of Dr. DeBakey's admonition to have a purposeful life, as most of the papers were associated with important prostate cancer projects. So with the exception of sporadic Mexican food feasts, which are an absolute life necessity for us transplanted Texans, I calculated that our renewed eating, exercise and spiritual habits would keep us both hearty till age 100.

While dietary studies are not yet conclusive, evidence suggests that a diet low in fat and high in fiber might control or even reverse, the spread of prostate cancer. In a study of the effect of fat on mice, scientists were able to show that a 20-50% reduction in fat caused prostate cancer tumors to grow at a significantly slower rate than usual, with the tumors becoming smaller in some cases.

It also appears that the mineral, selenium, which acts as an antioxidant, can be a preventive measure for prostate cancer. While studying the affects of selenium supplements for skin cancer, scientists discovered that the research participants who took selenium developed fewer prostate cancers than others types of cancer. In fact, they developed two thirds fewer cancers than the men who were on a placebo. A study at Johns Hopkins showed that men with the lowest levels of selenium were more likely to develop prostate cancer than those with high levels of selenium. Other studies have demonstrated that men who live in areas with soil that is rich in selenium have fewer deaths from a number of cancers. One interesting data point about selenium is that its effect is fairly quick, indicating that a man might be able to start taking selenium later in life as a cancer prevention supplement.

The Selenium and Vitamin E Prevention Trial (SELECT) was launched recently and will be conducted in over 400 sites. The study will include 32,400 men, will cost $250 million and will take twelve years to complete. When it is concluded, we will know if these two dietary supplements can protect men against prostate cancer.

Another important dietary question that is being studied with regard to cancer in general is the role of certain other vitamins, such as A and C, that are thought to act as antioxidants. Antioxidants prevent the formation of ions that damage the DNA. Damage to the DNA, in turn, is believed to play a part in causing cancer. Therefore, some scientists are trying to find evidence that consuming enough of these vitamins, either in the food we eat or through supplements, may help reduce the risk of developing certain kinds types of cancer.

Even if there is no definitive evidence about the effect of particular diets on prostate cancer, there is an interesting parallel worth noting. In Japan, the incidence of clinical prostate cancer is very low; 4 per 100,000. However, when people of Japanese heritage move to the United States, they usually change their diet, which had been rich in soy and fish, in favor of adopting our relatively high fat diet. Within a generation, they have an incidence of prostate cancer almost equivalent to that of Americans. Although animal fat appears to be the culprit, it is possible that this phenomenon may be due to other presently unidentified environmental factors.

Another interesting dietary connection between food and prostate cancer is with tomatoes, not the red-ripe, juicy, fresh ones as one would expect, but cooked tomatoes or tomato-based products. Apparently, the association involves lycopenes, which can be absorbed better when tomatoes are cooked.

Dr. Ed Giovannuci and his colleagues at the Harvard School of Public Health indicated in their study that there appears to be a correlation between the consumption of cooked tomatoes and a decrease in prostate cancer. This connection was discovered as part of a very large survey of physicians who kept track of what they ate. In the review of this survey, it was evident that those who consumed the most lycopenes had the least amount of prostate cancer. Dick and I now eat far more tomato rich pasta sauce than in years past, which certainly is a better choice for Dick than his former penchant for "little sizzlers" and bratwurst. This theory sounded good to me since I am willing to try any positive suggestion backed by good science, good sense and yummy taste.

If you have trouble convincing the male in your family to adjust his diet, you might try an imaginative measure like the following one I used with my late husband, James. Although I have been told that I am a world-class nag, nagging gets old and is hard work. But if I hadn't nagged James to watch his diet, he would eat a pound of fudge or indulge in some other similar dietary time bomb. His compromised digestive track after pancreatic cancer surgery could not take such abuse, yet he seemed to drop his guard at times and dive into the forbidden foods with the ferocity of a starving lion. As a diabetic, I understood his yearnings, especially for fudge.

Instead of nagging him to follow the doctor's admonitions myself, I decided to be innovative and hired someone to pose as a representative from the "Hassle Nag Service." A friend could have played the part just well but I felt the scene would be funnier and more effective if James faced a perfect stranger. I sent the "nag" to his office, whereupon she recited my list of reminders to take his pills and the doctor's list of off-limits activities and foods. His laughter was reward enough for my effort. From then on, when he was pushing the limits of his condition, I would threaten to call 1-800-HAS-NAGS, and we would both howl with laughter. It was a wonderful way to encourage him to follow his doctor's orders.

Women are natural people motivators, and since following a good diet is part of a healthy regimen, most women can motivate their partners with more creative ways than nagging them to adhere to a healthy diet and follow other similar instructions for good health.

Interestingly, diet may play a part in the prostate cancer found in African Americans. Some researchers think a high consumption of fat may contribute to the fact that members of this population have one of the highest rates of prostate cancer in the world, and they are more likely to die from prostate cancer than their white counterparts. Winston Dyer, an extraordinary leader in the prostate cancer awareness movement in New York, is working diligently to see that the significant increase in incidence and death is being addressed through many programs to help the African American community overcome this imbalance.

In addition, Dr. Timothy Thompson and his colleagues at Baylor College of Medicine in Houston are studying a protein linked to the spread of prostate cancer, which might explain why African-American men often have a more aggressive form of the disease.

Certain occupations have an increased incidence rate for prostate cancer, too, including drug and chemical workers, painters, rubber workers and other professions whose members are exposed to a number of toxins. Surprisingly, farmers also fall in this group, most likely because of their years of exposure to herbicides and other agricultural chemicals.

It appears that the incidence is also higher than normal for sedentary types like bookkeepers, whose prostates are confined to the seat of a chair all day. When I read this, I immediately pictured a group of inactive, desk bound executives hiding their prostates on the cushion of a swivel chair from 8-5, on a sofa from 7-10 and only letting them come up for air and sun on weekends between televised football games.

This theory is not too far fetched as investigators at the University of North Carolina have made an interesting connection between Vitamin D, the sunshine vitamin, and prostate cancer. In the United States, prostate cancer deaths are highest in the Northeast, which has less sun than in the lowest region, the sunny Southwest. Across the Atlantic, the deaths are highest in countries like Switzerland, Norway, Sweden and Iceland and lowest in sunnier countries like Italy. The parallel in this instance appears to be that the greater the amount of the sunlight, the lower the death rate from prostate cancer.

The speculation is that sunlight/ultraviolet light on the skin can increase Vitamin D levels that may prove protective. Very sunny Texas seems to be full of prostate cancer survivors, so it would be interesting to see if the Vitamin D/sunlight hypothesis holds up. If proven to be a factor, those men, who are now avoiding the sun to hold skin cancer at bay may be changing their travel plans to include the beach again to give their prostates some Vitamin D. It is important to note, that naturally occurring Vitamin D from the sunlight is not harmful, however, taking excessive doses of Vitamin D supplements can cause severe liver problems.

A few prostate cancer survivors blame their illness on their purportedly active sex lives. Actually, a few scientists have raised the hypothesis that excessive sexual activity and early sexual experience increases the incidence of prostate cancer because consistently sexually active men may have high levels of testosterone.

On the other hand, some hold that men with low sexual activity might be potentially more likely to have prostate cancer due to an accumulation of testosterone in the prostate from decreased ejaculation.

Neither of the theories related to sexual activity, however, has been confirmed by scientific data. Eventually, being able to determine their meaning may answer some extremely important questions about the role of hormones in prostate cancer.

Interestingly, the prevalence of prostate cancer varies widely from place to place and among ethnic groups, but the prevalence of microscopic/latent prostate cancer cells upon autopsy appear to be similar worldwide. In this vein, it is fascinating to note that one third of the men over 50, according to these autopsies, have latent prostate cancer cells. It is widely accepted that most men who are diagnosed with prostate cancer, have had latent prostate cancer cells in their bodies for decades. These facts make one wonder what environmental factors precipitate the cells' transformation from latent to clinical status. We do know that the lifetime risk of a man in the United States being diagnosed with clinical prostate cancer is about 15%. Fortunately, the PSA test does not usually "see" latent prostate cancer cells, since there is no indication that latent cells should be treated.

# 5.

## A Family Affair

When it appeared that our relationship was going to lead to marriage, Dick thought it was essential to apprise me of what I would be facing as the wife of a prostate cancer survivor, including the side effects from his surgery. Little did he know that he should have been more concerned about what he would be facing when he married me rather than the other way around. The truth came out during our pre-marriage counseling when the pastor asked me what I would bring to the marriage. "Chaos!" I said unfalteringly. I lived up to my promise. Dick's once peaceful, studious life is now filled with hordes of marvelous extroverts, constant commotion, exercise programs, my awful cooking and a huge mean cat, who gives no quarter to Dick's two dogs.

He also happily found himself a father and grandfather of girls for the first time in the persons of Lelia, my beautiful, extraordinary daughter and Elizabeth Grace, my cherubic granddaughter. Brent, our son-in-law, was a terrific addition to Dick's three sons, Rex, Dwight and Roger and his grandson, D.W. I appreciated the fact that our respective families were very kind to the two of us. This is often not the case when a father or mother remarries, but we were blessed with a supportive family on both sides.

Dick also brought his own heightened measure of activity, which basically centered on his now departed, chestnut shaped prostate—may it rest in peace. Before meeting Dick, I had heard of a prostate but was not quite sure of its exact location or function. The closest I ever came to the word was when I sang "let angels prostrate fall" in the familiar hymn. Now I was involved in a household where the prostate reigned supreme, at least in conversation.

Fortunately, I could comprehend his medical jargon and converse fairly well on the basics of prostate cancer, particularly after my mini-medical school experience. Like Dick, I had become medically knowledgeable the hard way. In my case, I was diagnosed years ago with acute intermittent porphyria, a rare, life threatening genetic illness. During my initial treatment at the National Institutes of Health, I spent months reading everything I could find on the disease and spent countless hours in their medical library trying to locate the best specialists in the country. As with prostate cancer a decade ago, there was little information for laymen, which made the search very difficult. However, I was able to confirm which physicians were the most highly recommended specialists in the field. I contacted the ones who were treating other porphyria patients or who were involved in clinical research, and I learned about the work they were doing. Finally, I met with a wonderful specialist, Dr. Karl Anderson at Rockefeller University Hospital in New York and became one of his research patients. He and his colleagues studied several experimental treatments before they discovered the one that saved my life.

After years of hospitalizations and experimental treatments, I was able to live without the threat of an early death and painful episodes hounding me. I used my newly found energy and grateful spirit to serve as the executive director of the American Porphyria Foundation and have continued in this voluntary position for twenty years.

My next step in gaining unsolicited medical knowledge came about when my deceased husband, James Lyon, was diagnosed with pancreatic cancer. James had had a problem with ulcers for many years. When he began having abdominal pain, he assumed that the ulcers were bothersome again and scheduled a visit with the gastroenterologist. I drove him to the doctor where instead of receiving treatment for the ulcers, we heard the devastating report that James had pancreatic cancer and might not survive more than a few months. We were overwhelmed with the staggering news.

Providentially, James lived three happy years instead of the usual six-month onslaught suffered by most pancreatic cancer patients. After his death, I took a hiatus from the world, as I was overcome with grief and not able to cope with more than simple daily living. The devastation I felt after his death propelled me to join the war on cancer. I may be just a foot soldier in this war, but my zeal is commando quality.

My enlistment in the war started with the premise that cancer is my enemy. Simple basal cell skin cancer that can be easily removed at a dermatologist's office is my enemy. Prostate cancer is my enemy. It can lie quietly for years or launch an assault so aggressive that it causes excruciating pain, breaks bones and brings a man to an untimely death. All cancers are my enemy, so I rejoice in the many major advances over this adversary that have occurred in recent years.

I liken cancer to an evil genius, who when facing a barrier, finds new ways to destroy it or stealthily go around it. For example, in prostate cancer, the cancer cell hangs on tightly to the prostate, but when it decides to forge ahead to a distant place, it first hits the very hostile environment of the blood stream. The blood vessels are smooth like tightly tiled walls with no visible hooks to which a cancer cell might attach itself. But when it does find a place to grab hold, the cell immediately sends out a signal that enables it to creep through the vessel walls. Next, it sends a message for the tissue to soften so that a new blood vessel can form. Then the cancer sets up shop and starts to multiply and becomes an ever more formidable foe.

Dick's reaction to cancer was similar to mine. Prostate cancer presented him with an educational opportunity he would have chosen to gain some other way. But having been treated successfully, he joined the war with the same measure of zeal as mine. This common commitment was the initial ground upon which we built a solid friendship, which eventually became a strong marriage.

Since Dick believes in obtaining an early benchmark PSA, he gave his sons two presents for their fortieth birthdays. Their first gift was a PSA test, paid in full. After they had the PSA test, they received a present of a more traditional nature: a big birthday check. The good news is that all of three his sons reported that their PSA's were in the lower end of the normal range. This was a case where bribery was legal and beneficial.

It is now widely accepted that there is a family link to prostate cancer. Approximately 25% of the men diagnosed with prostate cancer have a family history of the disease, indicating a hereditary influence. About 9% of the men with prostate cancer have one of the mutated genes that potentially increase their chance of developing hereditary prostate cancer, a purely genetic form of the disease that seems to occur at an earlier age.

The chance of a son's being diagnosed with the disease doubles after his father is diagnosed with prostate cancer, particularly if the father is diagnosed before age sixty-five. This genetic propensity can arise from either the father's or the mother's side of the family. The same risk holds true if a brother or a "blood uncle" is diagnosed and increases 8-11 times if two "first degree relatives" develop the disease. This risk increases with the numbers of relatives who have the disease.

Research on the family link has been limited, perhaps, because of the concentration in the past on the relationship between old age and prostate cancer. This inherited predisposition was recognized thirty years ago when a group of genealogists noted that prostate cancer appeared in family "clusters" and that these clusters were more prevalent in prostate cancer than in breast cancer.

Almost half of the prostate cancer diagnosed in men under the age of fifty-five, appears to be related to inheritance. Since this is the case, some people have asked about genetic testing. Unfortunately, none is available yet, however, scientists know the general area of the genes involved and are working on greater specificity.

If there is a family link, it is suggested that men be screened for prostate cancer starting at age forty-five, rather than the usual screening guideline of age fifty. Men who have first-degree relatives with prostate cancer should begin testing at age forty.

As a wife or sister or aunt or loving partner, you can help save your husbands and sons and nephews or other male family members by insisting that they have a PSA test and a digital rectal exam to keep this cancer at bay.

# 6.

## His Tale, No Pun Intended

**A** DRE is important to early detection as seen in the early detection recommendations of the American Urological Association:

> "Annual digital rectal examination (DRE) and serum prostate specific antigen (PSA) measurement substantially increase the early detection of prostate cancer. These tests are most appropriate for male patients 50 years of age or older and for those 40 or older who are at high risk, including those of African-American descent and those with a family history of prostate cancer. Patients in these age and risk groups should be given information about these tests and should be given the option to participate in screening or early detection programs. PSA testing should continue in a healthy male who has a life expectancy of ten years or more."

The American Cancer Society Prostate Cancer Screening guidelines are as follows:

> "Beginning at age 50, all men who have at least a 10 year life expectancy should be offered both the PSA blood test and a digital rectal exam. Men in high-risk groups, such as African Americans, men with close family members (fathers, brothers, or sons) who have had prostate cancer diagnosed at a young age should begin testing at 45 years."

### *The Life Saving PSA and DRE*

After we had known each other a few months, I asked Dick to tell me in detail about his unexpected journey into the world of cancer. He began with the diagnostic process.

Dick had retired as President of Pennzoil and was busy expanding and writing about his collections of Tiffany, Handel and Pairpoint lamps; mechanical musical instruments; Victorian silver; Wurlitzer jukeboxes; slot machines and rare antique fans. All of this changed one morning when he was listening to the radio. The announcer was telling the audience about the new PSA blood test, which measures the level of a specific protein in the blood, **prostatic specific antigen** (PSA for short), that is generated only by prostatic tissue and was being used as a marker to help detect prostate cancer.

Dick took note as the announcer explained that the PSA is a prostate specific test not a cancer specific test. In other words, a higher than normal PSA does not necessarily indicate cancer; rather it can indicate the presence of prostatic disease, prostate enlargement, infection or prostate cancer. However, cancerous prostate tissue secretes approximately 10 times as much PSA as normal tissue, so it is a good indicator of prostate cancer, particularly at higher levels or if it is increasing quickly.

Most of the PSA is located in the small tubes, which store semen, that run throughout the prostate. However, small amounts leak into the bloodstream and can be measured with the PSA blood test. A man's chance of having prostate cancer increases as the PSA level increases.

As a rule, when levels of PSA are higher than the normal reference range of 0-4, it can indicate that a man has prostate cancer, although further tests are needed to determine the diagnosis.

Having a PSA of 4 or less does not necessarily mean that a man is free of prostate cancer, but there are ways to sort this out over time. A PSA between 4 and 10 does not mean the man has prostate cancer, but it does require additional tests. However, levels of PSA above 4 indicate a 25-35% risk that prostate cancer will be found on a biopsy. Having a PSA above 10 is quite likely to indicate clinical prostate cancer and will almost always result in a biopsy.

By testing a patient annually and noting the change in the PSA, physicians can detect a potential cancer or a recurrence of the disease following treatment. Interestingly, prostate cancer is the most diagnosed cancer in America aside from simple basal cell skin cancers. Since the risk of prostate cancer, like breast cancer, is cumulative with age, the number of men being diagnosed will increase with time, absent effective prevention techniques.

If the PSA is above the normal reference range of 0-4 or if it has been escalating more than ¾ of a point in a year, a visit to a urologist is in order to determine the specific reason for the elevation. (It may be important to abstain from sex and a digital rectal exam prior to the PSA as both can increase the reading.) The urologist may rule out infection and rerun the PSA or perform further tests to determine and treat the problem once it is identified. One of the criticisms of the PSA is that it is not specific enough to keep men from undergoing additional unnecessary tests. Undergoing tests, however, is a small price to pay to discover cancer early enough to be cured, as Dick soon came to learn first hand.

During his routine physical, Dick mentioned the radio announcement about the PSA test to his internist and requested that she include it in his blood screen. The doctor agreed and admitted that this was the first PSA she had ever ordered. When the result came back at 4.2, only slightly above the normal reference range, the internist wisely referred Dick to a urologist.

When he arrived at the urologist's office, Dick was only mildly concerned, particularly since his PSA was so near the normal range, and he was not having any symptoms.

Unfortunately, many men forego medical tests because they have no symptoms. This is a mistake with prostate cancer, because a man generally does not experience symptoms until the disease is advanced. For this reason, prostate cancer is sometimes called the "silent killer."

Sometimes a man has mild symptoms, which are easy to ignore. When the symptoms, like bone pain, become severe, it is often too late to achieve a cure. In most instances, however, it is not too late to start treatments that will prolong life. This is why it is so important to convince your partner to have his PSA test. This one test has reduced the time for diagnosis of prostate cancer to five years earlier than was possible before the PSA test. Prior to the advent of the PSA test, men were diagnosed when the cancer became so large it could be felt during the DRE. By the time the cancer could be felt, it was often too late for the patient to be cured. Fortunately, that situation has changed considerably, primarily because of the early detection capability of the PSA test.

At that time, Dick was unaware of the silent nature of the disease, so he was not concerned as filled out the usual forms and checked "no" on the list of possible prostate-related symptoms:

- A feeling that the bladder has not emptied
- An interrupted or weaker than normal urine flow
- A need to urinate frequently
- Pain or a burning sensation during urination
- A problem starting or stopping urination
- Blood in the semen or urine
- Pain in the hips, kidneys, thighs, lower back or upon ejaculation
- Hesitancy or difficulty in starting urination
- *Nocturia* or being awakened to urinate during the night
- Inability to urinate in spite of the pressure to do so

Dick was proud of his overall good health and lack of checks on the urologist's symptoms list. After a short discussion with his new patient, the urologist promptly prepared Dick for a digital rectal exam (DRE). Dick had undergone this test many times. Before the development of the PSA blood test, the DRE was the primary screening test for prostate cancer and is still an important investigative procedure. It is an inclusive test as it allows the doctor to check for rectal cancer as well. For twenty years of these tests,

Dick's physicians had monitored a ridge on his prostate that was stable and benign, which also gave him additional assurance that all was well.

A urologist performs the procedure by lubricating his gloved hand and inserting a finger into the rectum to check for any abnormal or irregular firm areas which can indicate prostate cancer. After properly positioning the patient, the doctor is able to feel the rear of the prostate through the tissue lining of the rectum. Normal prostate tissue feels much like the tip of your nose, whereas cancerous tissue feels like the hard bridge of your nose. Cancerous tissue can also feel rippled or corrugated instead of smooth like normal prostate tissue. The results of the DRE are not clear-cut, however, because a tumor could be at the front of the prostate or be too small to feel or too inaccessible when a benign condition has caused the prostate to become enlarged.

Because the prostate is small and positioned deep in the body, patients are placed in the uncomfortable, awkward and embarrassing position of bending over the examination table for the DRE examination. Although the DRE is relatively quick, numerous men avoid having a DRE because of their fear of momentary discomfiture and embarrassment. I have discovered that men often call this procedure the "Dastardly Rectal Exam " or some other shorthand name like "the finger wave." By avoiding the DRE, these men risk not detecting a cancer at an early stage. (Although both the PSA and the DRE are important, if a patient insists on having only one, the PSA is the more important of the two tests.)

To illustrate, Hank Porterfield, the former chairman of US TOO! International, is an eight year prostate cancer survivor. As it so happened, Hank had been in excellent health most of his life except for a bout with polio when he was a young man. In the midst of his busy life managing his 300 real estate franchises, he developed high cholesterol, which led him to participate in a clinical trial to reduce the problem. Before, during and after the trial, he was required to have a physical, including a DRE. The results of the DRE were negative.

Shortly after the trial ended he took his annual trip to Florida for the winter and while there, he heard about the PSA test from his attorney who was undergoing treatment for prostate cancer. When he returned home, he asked his doctor to order a PSA, the results of which proved to be above the normal range. His subsequent biopsy indicated that he had prostate cancer. Armed with this news, he headed to an US TOO support group where he obtained a wealth of information, including the name of an exceptional surgeon. The PSA saved his life, so out of gratitude, he became involved with US TOO at the local level and has gone on to become the national leader of this support group network with 500 chapters.

I have always found it confounding that males speak of the DRE in torturous terms, yet women calmly endure pap smears, pelvic exams, mammograms and then the ultimate surprise from time immemorial: labor pains followed by the not so easy delivery of a precious baby. I dare say these examinations and childbirth are more difficult than a DRE but mentioning the comparison does nothing to encourage men to schedule one with their urologists.

One year during the Christmas season, I wrote a mini-play called *Coldfinger*, to the cadence of *The Night Before Christmas*. This was my attempt to make fun of the complaints of the male gender about the DRE. Dick and I were having a dinner party in honor of one of the actors who played James Bond in several of the 007 movies. Since he was also a prostate cancer survivor, we thought it would be amusing to have the "world premier" of my new *Coldfinger* play as our after dinner entertainment. The timing was especially momentous when we realized that most of the other males on our guest list happened to be prostate cancer survivors as well. As it turned out, several other guests were diagnosed at a later date, but fortunately, they did not develop the cancer as a result of my dreadful cooking that night.

*Coldfinger* was certainly not the usual coffee time entertainment, but then nothing is usual after cancer enters the scene. I can assure you that the play and the post dinner repartee were rollicking good fun.

Before the presentation, I jokingly introduced our aforementioned friend, Dr. Andrew von Eschenbach, as the play's special medical advisor and as the Chief Coldfinger of M.D. Anderson Cancer Center. It was my hope that he would lend some credible "hands on experience" to our upcoming spoof. Another close friend and prostate cancer survivor, Tom Redmond, an entrepreneur who made his fortune with his Aussie hair care company, played the villainous Coldfinger, and Cher Redmond assumed the role of the ever-sexy Bond girl, Loosey Goosey. One of Houston's most glamorous hostesses, Sandra Di Portanova, donned a physician's white coat, gathered a huge set of pliers, a saw and some other scary tools from Dick's workshop and took her place on our make-shift stage, as the infamous urologist, Dr. Barbarian. Dick had the honor of playing 007 while I narrated the play. The group howled with laughter and proved that night that "laughter is the best medicine."

### Coldfinger

*'Twas the night before Christmas*
*When all through the house*
*Not a creature was stirring, not even a mouse.*
*The reason was terror. Why no one would linger*
*Was fear of the vile Dr. Coldfinger.*
*All men were quaking since his ultimate mission*
*Was to do digital rectals without their permission.*
*Coldfinger was posing as a leading physician*
*But his goal was to put men in the "bend down" position.*

*This wasn't his only villainous objective*
*He planned to kidnap a beauty, for his mind was defective.*

*Loosey Goosey, a virginal, bosomy broad,*
*Was the target of his most devious fraud.*
*He viciously grabbed her, but like an act from heaven,*
*Who should arrive but the great 007.*

*Bond fought and subdued this most wretched brute*
*And dragged him to Dr. Barbarian in his birthday suit.*
*Then what to our wondering ears did we hear*
*But Coldfinger screaming in mortified fear.*
*"No, no," cried the villain, "nothing is worse*
*Than a DRE, the male's dreaded curse."*

*Bond made him endure Dr. Barbarian's exam,*
*And Coldfinger became as meek as a lamb.*
*Then Bond noticed his finger and stripped off the sheath*
*To discover a Goldfinger hidden beneath.*

*Though Bond saved the world from Goldfinger that night,*
*We're still left with Coldfingers instilling great fright.*

## Diagnostic Tests and Tools

### The TRUS and Biopsy

Even though Dick's PSA was only 4 .2 and his DRE was negative, the doctor ordered a transrectal ultrasound (**TRUS**). A TRUS involves placing a probe in the rectum to image the prostate using high-frequency sound waves and creating the image on a video screen. This ultrasonic imaging does not rule out cancer, but it can help locate suspicious areas within the prostate and determine the approximate size of the prostate. Knowing the size is essential to determine PSA density, which is the value of the PSA divided by the volume of the prostate. Determining the PSA density is a technique to help distinguish between benign disease and cancer. Essentially, the main function of the TRUS is to guide the biopsy needles.

While Dick's urologist was watching the ultrasound screen, he commented that the TRUS appeared clear and suggested that since the TRUS probe was already in place, it would be a good time to proceed with a **biopsy** and Dick agreed.

Guided by the image on the video screen, a spring-loaded, hollow biopsy needle was then inserted into the prostate through the rectum to obtain small "cores" of tissue about a millimeter in diameter. Dick was awake while the doctor took six samples or cores, three samples per side. In fact, he could watch the whole procedure on a television monitor. Current practice is to take up to twice as many samples. Some men have a little discomfort with the procedure, and others find it quite uncomfortable. Dick described the feeling like a mild bee sting that intensified with each shot. The pain is not from the rectum but is caused by the needle piercing the prostate.

Because of the added cost of sedation and its respective risk factors, most procedures are done without pain sedation. Since some men consider the biopsy to be very painful, there are a few steps that can be taken to lessen the discomfort, including lubricating the probe with anesthetic jelly. Prostate biopsies are now often performed under local anesthesia by infiltrating around the base of the prostate with lidocaine.

Because the biopsy needles pierce the wall of the rectum, an enema is given prior to the procedure and oral antibiotics are given before and after the biopsy to prevent infection. Patients are asked to stop taking aspirin or any blood thinning medications a week before the scheduled biopsy, but there are no dietary restrictions for the procedure and no restrictions for scheduled medications other than those that thin the blood. The biopsy takes about thirty minutes and after the biopsy is over, there may be a little blood in the urine off and on during the day of the procedure. All things considered, it is a relatively simple procedure.

What has been worrisome to some men is whether the biopsy can spread the cancer or help it escape the prostate along the biopsy track. At present there is no evidence of this, particularly considering the vast number of biopsies given for all kinds of cancers. Even if a few cancer cells escape into the bloodstream, they cannot survive, at least until they have developed metastatic capability.

Since the biopsies are relatively small samples of the total prostate, the cancer could be in locations other than those sampled. In other words, the results may be negative even though the patient has prostate cancer. In this case, it may be necessary to repeat the procedure at a later date. It is not uncommon to have a "false negative" biopsy (PSA less than 4) and later find cancer. That is why it is very important to repeat biopsies at intervals specified by the urologist and to follow through on subsequent biopsies if they are necessary.

I have heard that the whole biopsy process is like sticking a needle into a kiwi berry that only has a few black spots. Since the spots are tiny and are sometimes in places where they are not usually located, the needle can miss them entirely. The same holds true for a cancer biopsy, but nonetheless, the cancer is typically found through a biopsy.

One of Dick's best friends, Bill Douglass, has the reverse situation. When his PSA rose far above normal, he had his first biopsy and fortunately, all was well. On successive PSA's, the levels remained the same or increased several points. After each of these high results, he was given another biopsy. Thirty-two biopsies later, Bill still shows no sign of cancer on his slides. If he were not using such a reputable doctor, we would wonder if he was getting good medical care. However, his physician is excellent as is the hospital laboratory that does the pathology. Because of his large number of biopsies, we have often kidded Bill that he was acquiring a radical prostatectomy from the inside out, one needle at a time.

### The Gleason Score

Two of Dick's six biopsy samples were positive, both of which were on the left side. His **Gleason score** was also noted in the laboratory report. Prognostically, this is a very important number. These scores are pathology results of a grading system developed by Dr. Donald Gleason, the reference pathologist for the Veterans Cooperative Group. It is used to measure the aggressiveness of the tumor by looking at glandular patterns under a microscope.

Normal glands are quite uniform in appearance with a normal layer of two cells. The cancerous glands have a single layer of cells and become more and more irregular and disorganized until they are a mishmash of diseased looking cells. When the pathologists study the different biopsy samples, they see different patterns in different parts of the prostate.

Until Dr. Gleason described five specific categories or "grades" of such tumor patterns, they had difficulty classifying the cancer. Basically, the system is used to rank cell differentiation or the measure of distinction of the borders and architecture of the cell.

Grade 1 glands are well organized/differentiated in appearance and look almost like benign tissue. This grade is very rare, since the cells in most tumors have progressed beyond this level before they can be detected by the DRE or PSA. Grade 5 glands are so poorly organized that they are uniform sheets of cells with no glandular organization and are basically swirly in appearance. Fortunately, Grade 5's are quite rare, because the tumor is usually diagnosed before they reach this level. Interestingly, the higher the Gleason grade the less PSA the cells generate. As one would expect, a Gleason grade of three is the one most commonly found.

To determine the Gleason score, the pathologist finds the tumor with the highest volume in the needles and gives it a grade of 1 to 5. Then the tumor with the second highest volume is determined and given a score of 1 to 5. The Gleason score is the sum of the two grades. If just one tumor is found, the grade is doubled. So Gleason scores can range from two (1+1) to ten (5+5). The most common is six (3+3). There are many sevens (3+4 or 4+3). Sevens are significantly more aggressive than the sixes and the 4+3's are more aggressive than the 3+4's.

After the prostate has been removed, a more thorough examination of the cells can be can be performed. Not only can the Gleason score be determined more accurately, but the location and extent of the tumor can be also established quite precisely This information is called the pathologic stage of the tumor. The pathological Gleason score rarely declines from the clinical score but does often increase in about 25% of the cases.

The Gleason score is an extremely important number, since it indicates how aggressive the tumor might be. The differences between the scores are very significant. For example, a Gleason-6 tumor might be doubling every two to four years, while a Gleason-8 tumor might take two to four months and a Gleason-10 just two to four weeks.

Unfortunately, Dick's clinical Gleason score of 3+3 increased to 3+4 when the pathology on his prostate was completed. Also, instead of the cancer being found only in the left lobe, it was in both lobes of the prostate and had penetrated into the capsule on both sides but not through the capsule. His was definitely not the plain vanilla case he originally thought.

(Dick didn't learn all of this until many years after his surgery when he had the opportunity to review his slides with Dr. Tom Wheeler, chief pathologist at Methodist Hospital in Houston. Dick was also able to see that all of the cancer was in the lower part (apex) of his prostate on both sides.)

Also during this period, Dick requested that a DNA ploidy analysis be run on one of his tumor samples, which had been preserved at Methodist Hospital where his surgery was performed. This is a very sophisticated, expensive examination of the genetic composition of the tumor and is not run routinely as it generally correlates with the Gleason score. Dick's tumor was diploid, which meant that it had the normal pair of chromosomes. A worse result prognostically would have been tetraploid, double the normal number of chromosomes. Even worse is aneuploid, a very disorganized jumble of chromosome pieces.

These are not routine steps a man must have for diagnosis and follow-up after treatment. Dick asked that the extra pathology be performed as a matter of interest and education because he wanted to be well prepared for the questions he anticipated during his presentations on prostate cancer. It was also important to him to be able to talk about these tests if men who call him ask a particular question related to ploidy or other not so usual subjects.

## The Stage

Another very important, routine determination is the **Stage** of the cancer. **The Stage** is basically an assessment of the physical extent of the cancer defined by clinical results using the DRE, TRUS, biopsy, bone scans, CT scans, MRI etc. Staging is beneficial in determining the appropriate treatment for a specific case, because knowing the location and extent of the tumor allows the physicians to be more precise in their treatment recommendations.

Originally, an ABCD system, designed by Dr. Willett Whitmore from Memorial Sloan Kettering Cancer Center in New York, was used for staging classification. Today, however, the American Joint Committee/International Union Against Cancer has accepted the international TNM staging as the preferred system preferred. The T in the TNM staging is for the primary <u>Tumor</u> in the prostate. The N ranking characterizes the extent of lymph <u>Node</u> involvement, if any. The M ranking specifies whether a cancer has <u>Metastasized</u> beyond the lymph nodes.

Combining these three rankings gives physicians and patients a quick summary of the tumor and a more understandable guidance system to determine the best therapy for each patient. The T-N-M rankings have subsets of numbers and letters, which are even more definitive. For example, when the doctor says that his patient has a T3c-N2-MO, he will almost certainly suggest a different course of treatment than for someone with a T1c-NO-MO. Staging is done in two categories: clinical staging before treatment and pathological staging performed after the lymph nodes have been sampled and the prostate and seminal vesicles are removed.

Tumor rating

T0: There is no evidence of a tumor.

T1: Primary tumors cannot be detected with a DRE or TRUS.

T2: The tumor is confined within the prostate and is detectable with DRE and TRUS.

T3: The tumor extends through the capsule of the prostate. This is more dangerous than if it were contained within the prostate.

T4: The tumor has invaded other organs.

Node rating

N0: There is no lymph node involvement.

NX: The lymph nodes have not been assessed.

N1: The cancer can be found in one node in the area of the prostate.

N2: The cancer extends to multiple nodes.

N3: The cancer can be found in a mass not attached to the tumor.

N4: The cancer extends to multiple nodes in other areas of the body.

Metastasis rating

M-0: Metastasis is not detectable.

MX: Metastasis has not been assessed.

M1a: Evidence of the metastasis can be biochemically determined.

M1b: A single metastasis is located in a single site.

M1c: Multiple metastases are found in a single site.

M1d: Multiple metastases are found in multiple sites.

**The Partin Tables**

Another helpful diagnostic tool is the **Partin tables**, developed a number of years ago by Dr. Alan Partin at Johns

Hopkins. In addition to developing diagnostic tools, he also sees patients, performs prostate surgery and serves as the Editor-in-Chief of *Urology*, a leading medical journal.

By correlating things that are known before surgery--the patient's Gleason score, PSA value and the clinical stage of his cancer--an estimate can be made of the odds that the cancer is either contained within the prostate, has migrated outside the capsule, is in the seminal vesicles or has metastasized to the lymph nodes or beyond. In other words, the Partin tables can help men and their doctors predict the pathological stage of the tumor before treatment and then help them better determine the most effective course of treatment. The good news is that not only has there been a dramatic and favorable shift in the stage at presentation for men who are newly diagnosed with prostate cancer, but there has also been a migration within stages towards more favorable projected outcomes.

The Partin Tables were updated in 2001 to recognize these changes.  Again, it is important to remember that these tables are statistical indicators, not absolute guarantees.

### The Kattan Formula

Since characterizing the exact nature of cancers is very important, analytical tools are extremely valuable. A relatively new prognostic tool has been developed by Dr. Michael Kattan, a researcher at Memorial Sloan-Kettering Cancer Center in New York. His specialty is medical informatics; the use of artificial-intelligence techniques to predict outcomes in complex systems.

Using information from a large group of prostate cancer patients, Dr. Kattan developed a computer-based nomogram to predict how particular prostate cancer tumors will probably behave as they progress over time. This **Kattan Formula** can even be conveniently placed on a hand held Palm Pilot computer. Factors, such as a man's PSA, the stage of his tumor and his biopsy results are entered into the program.

With the press of a button, the nomogram calculates the probabilities of the five-year biochemical recurrence (as indicated by newly elevated PSA) of prostate cancer after primary treatment. Recently, a study of more than 4,000 patient records demonstrated that the nomogram predictions were remarkably close to the actual patient outcomes.

Essentially, the information derived from the nomogram can help a patient and his doctor decide whether treatment or monitoring is in order or how aggressive the treatment should be if it is needed. Scientists can also use this data to predict which patients can be helped by a specific clinical trial and use it to help assign patients to high-risk or low-risk groups.

These stages, grades and tables reflect a "statistical probability" and are not absolutely predictive for a specific individual because of a margin of error. Nonetheless, they are weighty building blocks to help a man make one of the most important decisions of his lifetime: how to treat his particular prostate cancer.

## *The Diagnosis*

Dick and his late wife, Charlotte, were absolutely stunned when they learned that he had prostate cancer. Couples react differently when they hear the prostate cancer news, even those who are prepared for such a diagnosis. Most are overwhelmed like Dick and Charlotte and find themselves less able to deal with the important decisions and practical issues ahead of them when they are in the most need of the capacity to do so. More often than not, men and women are also so bewildered by the diagnosis that they cannot remember much of their conversation with the physician after the cancer diagnosis is given.

This is why it is so very important to take notes during the visit with the doctor and to have pertinent questions prepared before each visit. Moreover, it is best to do these things in person as opposed to handing your list to the doctor for his written answers. Since many men are not apt to communicate their questions or relate more than their most basic symptoms, even to their physician, a woman can be particularly helpful by writing down her partner's symptoms and preparing questions ahead of time. Having been pre-warned that this can happen, some patients tape the dialogue in the doctor's office to insure that they heard the doctor correctly.

The following is a list of frequently asked questions. The two of you will have many more questions, especially those which are pertinent to your case.

- What do the results mean?
- What treatments are available and how effective are they for our particular case?
- What if the cancer has spread beyond my prostate? Is it still curable?
- What treatment does the doctor recommend?
- What are the risks involved?
- Does the doctor perform the recommended treatment and, if so, how often?
- How much time can we take to make a treatment decision?
- Who does the doctor recommend for a second opinion?
- Are there any dietary recommendations or restrictions before and after treatment?
- What are the physical and emotional side effects of each treatment, and how are they managed?
- What are the time expectations for the treatment, hospitalization stay and the recovery?
- How serious is his case in light of his particular health conditions?
- How advanced is the cancer?
- Are there informational brochures, books, video or audiotapes that we should procure?
- How much does testing and treatment cost and is the cost covered by Medicare and other insurance policies?
- Where can "we" find information about support groups?

- How can "we" find out about alternative medicines?
- What do "we" do next?

In 1991, Dick suddenly found himself among the 120,000 men being diagnosed that year, a number that has now increased to approximately 200,000. He and Charlotte faced the first question each of these other men and their families faced after diagnosis, "What do we do next?" I intentionally mention "we" because loving partners should both play a role in this educational and decision making process. Whereas, "What do we do next?" is the question all cancer patients face, it is generally a simpler question to answer with other cancers than with prostate cancer, because sufficient randomized trails have not been completed to give definitive answers about the efficacy of each treatment. Therefore, the decision requires a great deal of independent study of the treatment options, as well as lengthy discussions with a urologist, radiation oncologist, and, at times, a medical oncologist as well as other survivors. Weighing the options against a man's attitude toward specific treatments and specific needs is of particular importance. Even then, determining the best therapy is still difficult because there are still opposing viewpoints among the medical community about issues ranging from the need for screening to which treatment is best under a specific set of conditions.

Although gaining understanding about prostate cancer and the effectiveness of his specific treatment can help predict health difficulties, it still cannot protect a man from the uncertainties of cancer. Faith, family support, a strong body, great nutritional habits, and other positive factors are important as well. Plus, input from experienced mental health professionals and pastors can provide excellent guidance during the trying times.

At the time of Dick's diagnosis, patient information was almost nonexistent, so he wasn't aware of the many questions he should have asked his doctor. Usually, Dick studies things that interest him, but sadly, there were no books or brochures for laymen on prostate cancer available at the time of his diagnosis. Moreover, as far as he and Charlotte could remember, there was no one among their friends who had the disease with whom they could discuss their new problem. As it turned out, a groomsman in Dick and Charlotte's wedding had been treated successfully ten years earlier with radiation, the treatment of choice at that time. In forgetting their friend's case, they missed an opportunity to be infused with hope and first hand knowledge.

Although more than 30,000 men were dying annually of prostate cancer in the early 1990's, they seldom discussed the disease, particularly in mixed company. At that time, it was an almost invisible disease. In fact, an American Medical Association survey taken during that period revealed that forty-three percent of the participating doctors felt that many of their patients missed having timely prostate cancer treatment because of their inability to communicate about it. This is not news to females, who have dealt with man's propensity to "clam up" in times of extreme adversity from time immemorial. Fortunately, communication about the subject of prostate cancer has become much more open in the past few years.

Because they found themselves in this furtive atmosphere as well as in the midst of a medical information wasteland, Dick and Charlotte prepared for the worst. Still, Dick is a man whose middle name should have been "research," so it was surprising to learn that he had spent less time researching treatment options and treating physicians than he normally spent deciding on which new car to buy. The only reason, other than the information void, that he gives for this inconsistency in his nature is that he was in shock over the news of the cancer diagnosis and was operating at half speed.

I implicitly understood this. After each negative report on the status of his pancreatic cancer, James and I would be emotionally reeling, unable to think clearly. I can remember one instance when we had just received the news that an experimental treatment that had been holding the cancer back was no longer effective. Dr. Levine showed us the cancer "spots" on the x-ray. I could see the agony on his own face as he tried as compassionately as possible to advise us of the tragic news. Forlorn, James and I said nothing for a few minutes, but clung to each other trying to give one another strength. Then we began to discuss what we had just seen and heard. James talked about the implications of the metastasis throughout his lungs. In my subconscious desperation to minimize the tragic news, I could not remember seeing the many tiny "spots" of cancer sprinkled around his lungs. I only remembered seeing two tiny marks on the x-ray.

Generally, I was the one who paid close attention to everything the doctor said, made special notes of our conversations and stalwartly steeled myself in case we were confronted with a bad report. This time I was so overcome by the news that I was unable to put my thoughts together and tried not to collapse under the heavy emotional pain.

The first indication that we had been dreadfully traumatized occurred as soon as we exited the examining room. Although we had been to the clinic at least 200 times over the treatment years, neither of us could remember how to reach the elevators and had to ask the nurse for directions. We rode down to the lobby in doleful silence and headed to the car. As James and I walked out the front door of the clinic into the clammy, oven-hot Houston afternoon, we were shocked at the heat. We also faced another quandary. Neither one of us could remember where we had parked the car. Concerned about James' health, I walked him back into the cool lobby and situated him in a comfortable chair while I searched for the car. Since there were several large parking garages, it took the better part of an hour to find it. By the time we drove home, I was able to regain my composure and once again be the loving wife James needed.

Once I got James settled at home in a calmer state of mind, I handled his shots and medications and then addressed my own comfort needs. As always, I turned to the Lord, my daughter, Lelia, and my closest friend, Joanne in that order. If my own shoulder was to remain strong, I needed to be infused with their love, comfort and encouragement. This is important for all women who are in the "caregiver" role. A woman must not forget to care for her own spiritual, emotional and physical needs, lest her own strength and tenacity become depleted. If this happens, her ability to help her loved one will diminish while her stress level will rise exponentially.

It is astonishing how such stress can sometimes completely confound a person, even one who is accustomed to making complex decisions. When we most need to use good judgment, like after a cancer diagnosis, we are psychologically strapped and sometimes have the least ability to put facts together properly.

Again, that is why having both partners involved is so important. Two minds are better than one, and two genders are better than one. It is well established that men and women hear and understand things differently, so visiting the doctor with you partner can double your chances of absorbing what you heard during the visit and can decrease the confusion and anxiety surrounding your conversation.

In talking about the importance of having his wife, Ali, with him during important educational sessions or doctor's visits, Joe Torre said, "Ali and I are very lucky to have each other. One of the reasons we want to talk about the 'couples effect' of prostate cancer is to encourage men to work with their spouses in fighting this disease, not shut them out. After the diagnosis, there is a lot of information to absorb. I knew if I missed something, Ali would get it."

## Treatments

Although Dick and Charlotte did visit the doctor together, they were, nonetheless, heading toward a treatment decision without knowing about or taking advantage of the very limited resources that were available. Dick found himself in a perplexed state and did not take the best course to make a good decision. Instead he took Yogi Berra's not so wise admonition, "When you come to a fork in the road, take it." Dick set out down the path to choose a treatment without really thoroughly understanding the options. Neither he nor Charlotte even thought of making a list of questions to ask his doctor during their consultations about Dick's course of treatment, as patient interaction was not common at that time.

Having a prepared list of questions would have helped them when they met with the urologist. Nonetheless, they received from him a basic education on his treatment recommendation: a **radical prostatectomy**. He also prudently suggested that they obtain a second opinion in order to gain better insight into which treatment option to choose. It is also important to note that some insurance companies require a second opinion. However, most of the time, re-testing is not required since the original results can be forwarded to the second doctor.

Rather than consulting with a radiation oncologist, as he should have done in order to learn about a treatment other than surgery, Dick scheduled an appointment with another urologist, Dr. Richard Babaian, a well-known prostate cancer surgeon at M.D. Anderson Cancer Center. Dr. Babaian performed another DRE, reviewed Dick's test results and not surprisingly, agreed that he should have surgery.

Dr. Babaian is not only known for his surgical abilities, but he has also gained a reputation for his thorough DRE's. Dick told me that Dr. Babaian could find a tumor during a DRE even if it was on a man's tonsils. By the time Dick visited Dr. Babaian, he had endured at least 20 DRE'S over a number of years, so he felt like a veteran of the examination and could give a qualified assessment of any urologist's expertise in that area. From a patient's standpoint, irrespective of the discomfort, Dr. Babaian's skill at locating a tumor with a DRE should be greatly appreciated, because a thorough DRE can literally save a patient's life through early detection.

After the second surgical opinion, Dick returned to his original urologist, because he practiced at the hospital where Dick's past surgeries had been performed. In other words, Dick made his choice of surgeons dependent upon past medical procedures.

I have asked other men why they chose certain doctors and was surprised to hear that their selection was based on factors like geographical access, the size of the hospital room, a long standing friendship with the doctor, excellent hotels near the treatment center, etc. Sadly, one of my closest friends ignored the advice of one of the world's top cancer specialists and chose a doctor she met at a cocktail party, who was more charming than the specialist. This "charmer" was neither respected in the world of cancer in general nor was he a specialist in her type of cancer, but he had a winsome personality. She followed his rosy advice down a tragic path to a painful death.

The choice of the right surgeon is extremely important. Expertise and results are the most important factors to analyze when making this choice. It is not easy to acquire this information but asking the opinions and experiences of other patients and respected physicians is helpful.

Over time, Dick has set one pertinent criterion for the men who call him for information on prostate cancer surgeons. He suggests that they consider surgeons who perform at least 100 radical prostatectomies per year. He feels that his opinion was validated when this same suggestion was recently published in the Johns Hopkins prostate cancer newsletter. Expertise and results may not be related to the number of prostatectomies a surgeon performs, particularly if a very skilled surgeon is spending time teaching or researching and has kept his skills in tune, but checking the number of surgeries is a good starting place.

Another important issue is to determine the surgeon's success rate in preserving potency and continence. Unfortunately, it is almost impossible to obtain comparable information between surgeons, partly because few surgeons have the resources to keep accurate statistics.

There are many superb surgeons who are not one of the famous prostate cancer surgeons written about in books like this one. So it may not be necessary to travel to find the best one for your partner, but it is necessary to spend time and maybe money searching for the best. One factor which makes this easier to do today is that the hospital stays have been reduced from six or seven days to two or three days, so the time spent away from home is less than in the past.

When "interviewing" a surgeon, the following questions may be helpful to ask:

- How many radical prostatectomies does the surgeon perform each year?
- Is the surgeon board certified?
- Does the surgeon have a good record of preserving continence and potency?
- Where did the surgeon receive his training?
- Does the surgeon participate in training programs to enhance his technique?
- What are the surgeon's views on nerve sparing?

I realize the following analogy may sound trivial, especially in light of the importance of the surgical outcome, but when I see a good haircut, I immediately ask the name of the hairdresser and if she is consistent. Success speaks loudly.

Considering the number of radical prostatectomies a surgeon performs was a guiding determinant that Dick learned over time but didn't take into account after his own diagnosis.

Dick was very fortunate. Without thoroughly investigating the treatment options, without asking many questions of his physician, without talking to other prostate cancer survivors or even investigating other surgeons, Dick had a radical prostatectomy performed by a surgeon who, at that time, did not perform the operation often. Fortunately, his choice of surgery as his primary treatment was certainly the correct one for him. Although the end result proved that surgery was his best course of action, it was not undertaken as an educated decision. He is, however, very grateful to his urologist/surgeon for his persistence in finding the cancer and removing it in the nick of time.

Dick has been cancer free for eleven wonderful years. This, to him, was far more important when he made his treatment choice than being preoccupied with potential side effects and making compromises, which might risk curing the cancer.

The Radical Prostatectomy

A radical prostatectomy is one of the most difficult surgeries to perform. In that light, everything that can be done to make the surgery as effective as possible should be done in advance. This includes choosing an excellent surgeon, improving overall health and carefully following the doctor's orders

A radical prostatectomy is not performed until the inflammation and punctures in the wall of the rectum caused by the biopsy have had time to heal. The inflammation causes the prostate to adhere to the rectum. If surgery were performed before the inflammation heals, the surgeon might have difficulty separating the prostate from the rectum. This further complicates an already very complicated surgery and could mean that the surgeon might not be able to remove all of the cancer.

The goal of radical prostatectomy surgery is to completely remove the prostate, as well as the attached seminal vesicles. The surgery usually lasts two to three hours. Many men, like Dick, choose to donate their own blood prior to surgery to replace unexpected blood loss. This process entails giving one unit of blood each week for three weeks before the surgery is scheduled, taking iron prescribed by the doctor and refraining from blood thinning medications. Autologous donation today is rare, because much less blood is lost during surgery and the blood supply is of a better quality than in years past.

There are two surgical techniques: perineal and retropubic, which is the most common approach. With the retropubic method, the surgeon makes a mid-line incision from below the navel to the base of the penis. Most often, the surgeon next removes some of the pelvic lymph nodes and may send them to pathology where they are quick frozen with liquid nitrogen, then thinly sliced and examined for evidence of cancer. This specific biopsy is called a pelvic node dissection or a lymphadenectomy. The surgeon continues the operation if the frozen sections appear to be free of cancer and aborts the operation if they are positive. Some surgeons do not perform a "frozen section," particularly for the low-risk patients, rather they sample the nodes and have the nodes analyzed after the surgery is complete. They believe that removing the cancer is the best course of action regardless of whether metastasis to the nodes has occurred in order to keep men from suffering urinary complications when the cancer enlarges the prostate. Next the surgeon separates the prostate and the seminal vesicles from the bladder and the rectum.

After this has been accomplished, the entire prostate gland is removed by cutting through the urethra just above the external urethral sphincter, which is a voluntary sphincter comprised of striated or skeletal muscle, and by cutting just below the internal sphincter, which is an involuntary, smooth muscle at the bladder neck. Then the surgeon, using a Foley catheter as a guide, reattaches the urethra to the bladder neck with many very fine sutures in order to make the connection urine-tight. The catheter, which runs from the bladder out through the penis, remains in place for about two weeks following surgery in view of the fact that the patient is almost always incontinent during that period.

At one time, surgeons did not even know that the tiny nerves involved in erections were lying along both sides of the prostate, so they inadvertently cut them during the prostatectomy, thus leaving the man impotent. Now the picture has changed, and men are not automatically impotent after a prostatectomy. If nerve sparing is an option, the blood vessels are clamped and sutured in such a way that the surgical team can more clearly view the prostate and the surrounding area. It also enables the surgeon to see the two neurovascular bundles that are specific for an erection. These bundles are a network of blood vessels and nerves running along the outside of and adhering to the capsule of the prostate. It is difficult to separate the prostate while keeping either one or both of these tiny bundles intact.

Nerve sparing cannot be performed on all men. Because these tiny neurovascular bundles adhere to the surface of the prostate gland, they are not spared when there is a chance that the cancer could be nearby or on the nerves already. When at least one of the nerve bundles cannot be spared, complete impotence occurs. Unfortunately, even when the nerve sparing procedure is performed, some men still have impotence, but the numbers who benefit from the procedure are increasing.

Dr. Patrick Walsh, Chairman of the Department of Urology at Johns Hopkins in Baltimore, devised this technique in the late 1970's, when incontinence and impotence were prevalent side effects after a prostatectomy. First, prostate cancer surgery was exceptionally bloody, so much so that it affected the surgeons visibility during surgery. At that time, even suction tubes could not drain the area enough to keep up with the blood flow.

In turn, surgeons could hardly avoid cutting through the urethral sphincter, thus causing incontinence. Dr. Walsh changed this difficult situation by studying the blood flow patterns and devising a technique to clamp off the veins supplying the prostate area. This improvement diminished the blood supply during surgery, vastly improved visibility and reduced the need for transfusions.

Next he turned his attention to the problem of impotence. However, studying the prostate was difficult. Since cadavers were the source of anatomical studies, it was almost impossible to examine the prostate, because the prostate was enmeshed in fatty tissue, which was destroyed when the embalming process took place.

As it turned out, Dr. Walsh connected with Dr. Peter Donker, a retired Dutch urologist. Dr. Donker had studied the prostates of stillborn infants and discovered that the fatty tissue was thinner than normal, and the prostate nerves were larger. Walsh then made an important discovery. The nerve bundles responsible for an erection lay on the outside of the prostate and were connected to the prostate by a very thin layer of tissue. He surmised that, if it were possible to lift the tissue away from the prostate, damage to the nerve bundles could be minimized. As noted above, although using this technique has preserved the potency of many, many men, it has not been always been successful. Again, surgical expertise is vital. Also, there are other factors that affect potency, including the potency of a man prior to surgery, his age and the location of the tumor.

Dr. Walsh's significant contributions to diminish incontinence and impotence are greatly appreciated by hundreds of thousands of men, who have retained their potency and continence through his work on their behalf.

Unfortunately, despite efforts to spare these nerves during surgery, nerve damage still occurs. Since these nerves control blood flow to the penis, the damage causes erection problems in 50-80 percent of patients who have a radical prostatectomy. The potency effect of this surgery is related to the man's age, the extent of the nerve sparing that is possible, the skill of the surgeon or a combination of all of the factors.

Most often, men under 60 years old, who have strong erections before surgery, are usually the ones who recover fully functional erections.

Because of the trauma to these nerves, most men will not be able to get an erection during the first year after this surgery unless they use a medication or treatment. Later, some men will be able to achieve erections and others will continue to have difficulty. However, regardless of their potency, they will still be able to have an orgasm. The only difference is that there will not be any sperm, and it will be a dry orgasm.

Hope, however, springs eternal. Surgeons have pioneered a new nerve grafting technique to replace one or both of the nerves destroyed during the prostate surgery. The first nerve graft was performed in 1997 at Baylor College of Medicine in Houston by Dr. Peter Scardino, a urologist, and Dr. Rahul Nath, a plastic surgeon. Plastic surgeons, who are adept at reconstructive microsurgery, remove approximately a five-millimeter piece of the sural nerve, which runs along the ankle. This nerve is then grafted during the radical prostatectomy surgery. It usually takes up to two years to know for sure whether the graft has worked. During the first six months there is little response, if any, but erections can eventually return thereafter.

If patients, having only one nerve removed, are grafted, 75% of those who have not had chemotherapy or radiation regained their potency. If they have had prior therapy, the percentages decrease. Some institutions do not spare the nerves in any event because of the later risks of cancer recurrence, so they now perform nerve grafting.

After surgery, the prostate is examined by the pathologist to determine if the cancer was confined within the prostate capsule or has spread through the capsule into the surrounding pelvic cavity or to the seminal vesicles. The pathologist coats the outside of the prostate and the surrounding tissue with India ink. Then it is cut into 8-10 slices, mounted in paraffin blocks and placed in a preservative substance for twenty-four hours. Then ultra-thin slices are obtained, stained and carefully examined under a microscope. The ink creates boundaries to help the pathologist see where the scalpel cut. If the pathologist sees cancer cells at the edge of the India ink, then it is likely that the scalpel cut cancer, which means all the cancer was not removed. This is known as a positive surgical margin. If the pathologist sees that all the edges are clear of ink, it is likely that all of the cancer has been removed.

The radical prostatectomy is known as the gold standard of treatment. Most men choose to have a radical surgery as their best hope of eliminating the cancer, particularly if the cancer is confined within the prostate and the tumor is a low grade. Most men, who have cancer that is confined to the prostate or has even penetrated into the wall or capsule, have been cured. This is one reason scientists are trying to improve testing in order to determine if the prostate cancer is, in fact, confined. If all of the cancer is removed, no further treatment is needed. It is very important to understand that cancer is a very fierce foe and small measures usually do not eliminate it.

At the time of his diagnosis, Dick was younger and very physically fit, and his tumor was apparently confined to the prostate. He was the perfect candidate for a radical prostatectomy. Most surgeons agree that younger men are better surgical candidates, because of the long-term survival rate and the relative difficulty of the surgery.

Surgery is also sometimes performed to debulk the tumor even though nodal metastasis has occurred. Some physicians feel that debulking the tumor decreases the tumor burden, increases the effectiveness of hormonal treatment and avoids future urinary problems.

The most common surgical complications of the radical prostatectomy are excess bleeding and injuries to the rectum. Although only less than one percent of patients die during the surgery and only a few of them are under the age of sixty-five, it remains a more difficult, invasive treatment than radiation. The guideline is not to perform aggressive treatment such as surgery or radiation on men with a less than 10-year life expectancy due to age or co-morbidities.

When your partner arrives home from the hospital, it is important to watch that he has not formed blood clots in his legs causing extreme pain. Some doctors prescribe blood thinning medications or compression hose to prevent clots. Walking is also a very important measure to help prevent clots by pumping the blood back to the heart. Another preventive measure is to sit with your legs elevated, thus improving blood flow through the veins. Also, it helps to not sit upright in a chair for long periods of time. Notify the doctor immediately if you see any warning signs of a clot; pain and swelling in the leg or calf. Patients might even experience chest pain, coughing up blood, shortness of breath or fainting. These signs could indicate that a clot has moved into the lungs and could be life-threatening. It is common for a man to ignore these warnings, but hopefully, the woman in his life can overrule him in this regard and locate a physician as soon as possible, saving his life in the process.

Constriction at the bladder neck can also take place after surgery when scar tissue forms where the urethra and the bladder neck are sewn together. Although this does not occur frequently, you should be aware of the major symptom: a dribbling stream of urine when the bladder is full. If this is the case, contact the physician who can open the constriction and teach you how to keep the constriction open with a small catheter. As referred to earlier, the major side effects that can occur after surgery are incontinence and impotence. An entire chapter is devoted to each of these.

Generally, as we have said, aggressive treatment such as radiation or surgery is not performed on men with  less than a ten year life expectancy. However, one surgeon made an exception for the president of a middle-eastern country and performed a radical prostatectomy on him at age seventy-six. The decision to operate was definitely not based on the man's title, but rather the fact that he was in superb physical shape. It was rumored that he could still carry a machine gun twenty-five miles across hot, rugged territory, but that was probably more speculative than fact. However, after watching my own husband recently build a retaining wall with heavy railroad ties, use a jack-hammer to tear up part of a concrete driveway and then haul the slabs to the dump, I am not so sure that the desert trek was pure conjecture.

Conversely, there are plenty of fifty-year-old men who fit the age criteria but could not manage a two mile walk, suffer from hypertension, maintain a high-fat diet, smoke a few packs a day and are basically unhealthy. Perhaps, there needs to be another surgery determination category for the ageless Jack Lalanne types.

Radiation

Early prostate cancer can also be successfully treated with radiation therapy. Radiation destroys cancer cells by altering their capacity to reproduce or by inciting apoptosis, which is a self-destruction process causing cell death.

Radiation as a primary treatment tends to be the treatment choice for older men, because radiation may cure or retard their cancer and increase their life expectancy to the point that they can live a substantial number of years symptomatically unaffected by the disease. Those men who choose radiation also tend to have smaller tumors or a physical condition that precludes surgery, such as cardiovascular problems. If cancer has possibly spread into the pelvic area, radiation would be the treatment of choice. Like other treatments, radiation is not always curative, particularly with aggressive or widespread cancer. Nevertheless, it is a good option for men who prefer a less invasive treatment for any number of other reasons. The five-to-ten year survival rate is about the same as for surgery. However, it appears after the ten-year period, the survival rate of surgery patients surpasses that of those who have had radiation. Again, figures for surgery and radiation vary with the expertise of the surgeon and the radiation oncologist, plus a number of other factors.

As with surgery, it is important to select a radiation oncologist who performs a significant number of prostate treatments per year. Since oncologists tend to treat multiple organs more than urologists, you should ask the radiation oncologist how many prostate cancer treatments he or she has performed. It is also important to consider the reputation of the radiation department as a whole. A top cancer institution usually has the newest equipment and very experienced staff.

One form of radiotherapy is **external beam radiation**.

Usually, the course of treatment for this form of radiation is given in thirty-five to forty treatments, five days a week over a seven or eight week period. The weekend "off days" offer the patient a much needed rest and are also useful for another purpose. Benign cells can recover quicker than malignant cells so more of these benign cells survive with "off days."

The patient receives high energy x-rays from a linear accelerator over a broader area for the first five weeks followed by a "cone down" or more narrowed focus over the last two or three weeks of treatment. A physicist and a radiation oncologist determine the plan for the radiation field and a technician carries out the plan with the accelerator, which is computer controlled. The specifically determined plan is monitored over the course of the treatment.

With external beam radiation, the most recent technological development is the use of computers to visualize the prostate and seminal vesicles in a three dimensional simulation. This equipment enables the therapists to locate the prostate more exactly and place the radiation beam more precisely. The radiation therapist places lead-shielding blocks at the radiation beam aperture to protect non-cancerous tissue when the external radiation is applied and to focus the beam with more precision. This process called three-dimensional conformal therapy also lowers the incidence of future side effects from radiation. It is, therefore important to know what kind of simulation is being used and if true conformal radiation is available.

Radiation treatments are given in specially designed rooms. Although radiation therapists are not in the room during the treatment, they will be in an adjacent room watching the patient carefully on closed circuit television and communicating with the patient over an intercom system. During external beam radiation therapy, patients are not radioactive, so they need not take special precautions. Each radiation treatment lasts only a few minutes, and when the treatment is over, the patient is free to continue his normal activities.

Radiation can cause side effects, too, but they may not be immediate as with surgery. In fact, they can occur months or even years after the radiation. During the treatments, aside from incontinence and impotence, a man may experience a variety of other symptoms: fatigue, diarrhea with or without blood in the urine and stool, rectal pain and bowel frequency, urinary urgency, irritated intestines or bladder irritation. Some men do not have any symptoms for a few weeks after they begin receiving radiation treatment, but thereafter they have the above mentioned symptoms that vary in severity until a few days after the completion of the therapy. Interestingly, some men develop these symptoms long after their course of treatment

Some men chose radiation with the assumption that they have a better chance of sustaining potency than with surgery. Although erection problems are initially less common with radiation than with surgery, they are still frequent following radiation. Impotency appears to be about the same for both treatments but can be delayed for up to 18 months or so with radiation, because the cell damage occurs over a period of time rather than immediately as in the case of surgery.

Radiation affects a man's erection by damaging the arteries that carry blood to the penis and causing scar tissue near the prostate, which also reduces blood flow to the penis. As the irradiated tissue begins to heal, the internal tissue becomes scarred. The walls of the arteries lose their ability to expand so that blood can flow into the penis. Depending on the nature of the damage during radiation, some men can regain potency over a period of time. Incontinence is, however, another issue. The incidence of incontinence with radiation is less than with surgery.

**Proton beam therapy** is a lesser-known type of external beam radiation therapy, which is only performed at one center in California and one in Massachusetts. It will be performed at MDACC after their facility to house the machine is completed in a few years. It appears that proton beam therapy will be at least as effective as the conventional external beam radiation. The advantage of this type of beam is that its energy declines rapidly after it passes through the target. It remains to be seen if its ability to decay rapidly after hitting the target will be better for special applications such as treating prostate cancer, where it is important not to radiate surrounding organs such as the bladder and rectum. This type of therapy is significantly more expensive than conventional radiation treatments.

The second major form of radiotherapy is **brachy-therapy** which many men are now choosing as a primary treatment for prostate cancer, particularly if the tumor is small or at an early stage.

Brachytherapy, also known as interstitial radiation, internal radiation therapy or seed therapy, involves permanently implanting minute radioactive Palladium 103 or Iodine 125 "seeds" directly into the prostate using ultrasound guidance. These "seeds" continue to emit low-energy radiation for months until the radiation effect is complete and has, hopefully, destroyed the tumor. Although the seeds remain in the patient's body for life, their effect is time-limited, and they do not pose a threat to the patient's future health or anyone who is near them.

The advantage of this type of therapy is that the radioactive seeds can be placed accurately using ultrasound technology; thus delivering maximum radiation directly into or near the tumor and minimizing the damage to surrounding tissue. Another advantage is that the entire procedure can be completed in less than two hours on an outpatient basis, although some patients remain in the hospital for several days if complications become a potential problem.

Before having brachytherapy, a man should undergo a physical examination and have a cystoscope procedure to make sure there are no abnormalities in the prostate or that the cancer has not spread into the bladder. Then the patient has an ultrasound and CT scans. These procedures enable the doctor to determine the number of seeds needed, the exact location and depth to place each seed, depending on the strength of the radiation. Generally, a patient receives between fifty and eighty seeds depending upon the type of radioactive material used.

Several days before the procedure, it is suggested that the patient eat a low fiber diet. He is given a bowel cleansing preparation the night before the procedure and is asked to take an enema the next morning.

Before brachytherapy, the patient is given intravenous antibiotics and either general anesthesia or spinal or epidural anesthesia. Spinal anesthesia involves one small injection into the spinal fluid causing him to feel very numb from his waist to his feet. It is very important not to sit up in bed when the numbness is gone as sitting up too soon after spinal anesthesia can cause a terrible headache.

Epidural anesthesia involves having a small tube inserted at the small of the back into the vertebrae. An epidural anesthetic is injected through the tube thus numbing the nerves controlling the lower body. Unlike spinal anesthesia, this type of anesthesia can be given continuously, which enables the anesthesiologist to adjust the dosage, pain relief and numbness.

A radiation oncologist or urologist then inserts hollow needles containing the seeds through the perineum, which is the area between the rectum and the scrotum. The seeds are then guided into the prostate gland through the needle using ultrasound to visually place the seeds at specific locations. Then the needle is removed. This process has made the seeds potentially more successful than years ago when they were placed in the prostate by finger guidance, which was very imprecise.

After the procedure, patients are taken to a recovery room for a few hours where ice bags are placed between their legs to reduce the swelling. When the numbness has dissipated, the catheter is usually removed. You and your partner can then go home with a round of antibiotics, anti-inflammatory and pain medications. He should not drive for at least twenty-four hours after this procedure. In fact, some doctors will not perform the procedure if he does not have someone to accompany him home or has not made arrangements to stay in the hospital. In fact, most men are very fatigued for a period of time after the brachytherapy and need plenty of rest and a healthy diet.

Complications can occur with brachytherapy. Urinary retention, which is the inability to empty the bladder, is a major complication that generally improves after a week. This retention problem is due to inflammation and swelling caused by the trauma to the tissue around the implanted seeds. Some men also reported that they had bowel problems, other urinary problems and prostatitis. The complications of incontinence and impotence as well as other potential problems are discussed in their respective sections.

When the patient returns return home, the physician will provide a list of "do's and don'ts." This list should be followed carefully. Because some of the implanted radioactive "seeds" can leave the body in a man's urine, he will also be given a special lead container through which he should urinate to keep any "seeds" from being dispelled into the toilet. In this way, these "seeds" can be collected for proper disposal.

Although results obtained to date are promising, not enough evidence exists to determine the long-term curative effect of brachytherapy beyond ten years. It is also becoming apparent that high-risk cases (higher PSA, higher Gleason, larger prostates) require that brachytherapy be supplemented by a reduced dose of external beam radiation therapy. Furthermore, it is indicated in some circles that complications, particularly those involving the bowels, are higher with this combined therapy than with external beam radiation or brachytherapy alone. Impotence and incontinence appear to occur less often with brachytherapy, which may be another reason this therapy is gaining in popularity.

It is important to note that some recent studies have indicated that brachytherapy alone is less likely to eradicate the cancer than three-dimensional conformal external beam radiation or a radical prostatectomy.

As with surgery and radiation, experience and skill in performing brachytherapy are also of utmost importance.

### Cryotherapy

Cryotherapy or freezing of the prostate is a relatively easy, minimally invasive treatment option, but it has lost popularity as a treatment as the evidence mounts that the results are disappointing. Probes circulating liquid nitrogen are inserted through the perineum into the prostate in much the same way as needles with brachytherapy. The freezing process is monitored using ultrasound. To completely eradicate the tumor might require freezing the entire prostate, which would damage the urethra or the rectum.

This damage can be reduced by circulating warm liquid through the urethra; however, this process can also compromise the treatment. Again, more long-term data is needed to determine its effectiveness. Very few cryotherapy treatments are being performed today, because of reports that the cancer was not completely eradicated with this approach and the side effects, such as erectile dysfunction appear to be substantial.

Although ultrasound makes it possible to "see" the freezing process, doctors still lack uniformly accurate methods of measurement to be certain that sufficiently low temperatures were achieved to actually kill the cancer cells.

Hormonal Therapy

Hormonal therapy is a systematic approach used to control prostate cancer, whereas surgery and radiation are rifle shot therapies designed to remove or kill the cancer, respectively. The good news is that hormonal therapy almost always works. The bad news is that it is not a curative treatment and only works for a period of time, which varies between patients.

Hormonal therapy works by shutting down the production of testosterone, a male hormone, which "feeds" the prostate cancer. These hormones are androgens, thus the process is known as **androgen ablation** or **androgen deprivation**.

Hormonal therapy "starves" the androgen dependent cells, but does not kill all of the cancer cells, some of which are androgen independent at the outset and, thus, can continue to grow without androgens. Therefore, hormone therapy cannot be considered a curative therapy.

Although not a front line primary treatment, it is sometimes being used as a pre-treatment and a post treatment for radiation. Hormone therapy is also used as a stopgap treatment for men who have life expectancies of less than ten years due to their age or co-morbidities.

The primary use of hormonal therapy is to treat patients who are either incurable at diagnosis or who have had primary or adjuvant treatment failures: a rising PSA after surgery, radiation or both. As noted above, it is almost always successful in achieving significant reductions in PSA as the androgen dependent cells die. At the same point, ranging from six months to ten years or more, the PSA will start to rise again. Then, either an alternate form of hormonal therapy will be used or chemotherapy will be initiated.

Trials are underway to determine if hormonal therapy can be applied intermittently to reduce the length of time the patient suffers from the side effects, like loss of sexual drive, hot flashes, fatigue and osteoporosis. Preliminary results indicate that intermittent therapy may be as effective as continuous therapy. The hope is that it will be better, but that remains to be seen. If intermittent therapy turns out to be equally successful, the quality of life benefits are substantial since all of the side effects are reversible, except perhaps, osteoporosis.

The most widely used method of hormonal therapy is through monthly, quarterly or tri-annual injections of **leutenizing hormone-releasing hormone agonist** (LH-RH). The most commonly prescribed of these injections are Lupron (leuprolide) and Zoladex (goserelin), which are given every three to four months respectively to disrupt the very complex chemical messages upon which the production of testosterone depends. When a man first starts taking the LH-RH agonist, his testosterone levels increase dramatically. This "flare" occurs because the signal the LH-RH sends stimulates the production of LH. It takes about ten weeks before the testosterone levels decrease into the range of surgical castration. Since these drugs shut down testosterone production, a man's almost always loses his sex drive (libido), and he can experience hot flashes, fatigue, breast tenderness, breast enlargement, muscle loss and osteoporosis.

Osteoporosis is becoming more and more important, because men are being treated at an earlier age and surviving longer.

LH-RH treatments are very effective but are quite expensive, costing about six thousand dollars a year. However, these injections are administered by a doctor and, therefore, are covered by Medicare and most other insurance plans.

I personally know the power of LH-RH and was surprised when I heard that this was a prostate cancer therapy. When I was seriously ill with porphyria, my bouts with the disease were congruent with my menstrual cycle and ovulation. Strangely, I was given the same Lupron injections as men with prostate cancer take today, except the doses were smaller and given daily. These injections were used to stop my cycle and ovulations and, in turn, stop my related porphyria attacks. So when a group of prostate cancer survivors are in the midst of discussing their doses of LH-RH or it's side effects, I chime right into the conversation. I try to add my own commentary about my Lupron induced hot flashes, my terribly dry skin, my newly pooching tummy, my cranky disposition and my oh so many unjustified teary moments. The gals think it is funny, but the men do not see my remarks as any laughing matter. Nor do they like to have the LH-RH side effects identified as male menopause either.

I was glad to see our friend, Harold Burdine, inject some humor into this difficult subject. When Harold was placed on hormonal therapy, he sent the following email to his friends back home in Mississippi. His letter tells about his trip to M.D. Anderson Cancer Center in Houston and the steps that led him to the LH-RH hormonal treatment:

*I saw my new doctor, Dr. Andrew von Eschenbach, at MD Anderson Cancer Center (MDACC) for the first time at 9 AM on Wednesday morning. After viewing another ultrasound, he told me that the cancer had spread outside my prostate. At that time, he could not tell me just how far it had spread, but he did call it an "angry, aggressive one" and said that surgery was not an option at this time. He also said that it was unique. No surprise to Tomie and me, I have never done anything halfway.*

80

*Dr. von Eschenbach wanted me to visit with Dr Christopher Logothetis, a medical oncologist, who is one of the best in the country, but it usually takes weeks, if not months, if at all, to get an appointment with him. Dr. von Eschenbach then told me he had taken the liberty to call Dr. Logothetis on my behalf, and if I could rush over to his office within ten minutes, I would become one of his patients.*

*Each patient at MDACC is assigned a Patient Advocate upon entering the clinic and mine was Conner Burdine. We must be related because all of us Burdines descend from one Richard Burdyne, who packed up his croaker sack some time in the 1700's and hopped a boat to South Carolina. Conner helped me through the labyrinth of the hospital, and we made it to Dr. Logothetis' office in time. The doctor spoke with Tomie and me for a good while. I might add here that none of the doctors, nurses, staff, etc. at MDACC, talk to you, but with you.*

*Dr Logothetis said that he was concerned with the way the cancer had grown so rapidly and that I had a relatively low PSA reading given the size of the tumor. He ordered more tests, an EKG, another chest x-ray, and a bone marrow biopsy. I had heard horror stories about the bone marrow biopsy, but it was not so. The staff at the Bone Marrow Aspiration clinic at MD Anderson performs the procedure every fifteen minutes, 8 hours a day, five days week. Believe me, anyone who says they are painful did not have the procedure done at MD Anderson. On a scale of one to ten, with ten being a bad bee sting, this was at most a three or four.*

*Then came THE WAIT. Waiting for the biopsy results to come in was one of the longest three hours I have ever spent in my life, in fact, it felt more like six months. Dr. Logothetis called us in to the examining room and shared the good news that the cancer had not spread to my bone marrow or other organs and that it was not the very aggressive small cell carcinoma. This meant that I would be prescribed hormone shots, which will stop all testosterone production in my body. The nurse lovingly and kiddingly called the hormone therapy a payback to us men. Because I will be on these shots for some time, I will experience mood swings and hot flashes, so*

*I am giving everyone fair warning that I will be crabby once a month.*

*I may also have a series of chemo treatments in conjunction with the shots, which will be administered once a month anywhere I choose, even at home in Mississippi. There is the possibility that the tumor will shrink enough for surgical removal, so please pray, "Smaller, Smaller!"*

*Dr Logothetis told us to understand, "This is not a 100 yard dash anymore, but a marathon." Marathons are things Tomie and I can manage. He also said that ATTITUDE was everything. We can manage a good attitude, too.*

*So, there we are. There is no way I will ever be able to thank each and every one of you for your thoughts, good wishes, and most of all, your prayers.*

*God Bless you all, Harold*

It is not easy to muster up a good attitude when life throws you such a curve ball, but Harold and Tomie are a wonderful couple, who have managed to maintain an optimistic outlook and keep all of their friends and family smiling.

There are two components of hormonal therapy: **chemical castration** (LH-RH) and **surgical castration** (orchiectomy) both of which eliminate the testosterone produced by the testes. There is also the equivalent of testosterone produced by the adrenal glands. This process can be blocked by the use of antiandrogens, which are given in pill form. Antiandrogens work by blocking the testosterone from changing into dihydrotestosterone (DHT), which is what "feeds" the cancer. The most popular antiandrogens are **Eulexin** (flutamide) and **Casodex** (biclutamide), but they are also expensive, approximately $3000 a year. These agents are used in combination with LH-RH to achieve what is called a total androgen blockade. They are also used to mitigate the LH-RH-induced testosterone "flare." Using it as a pre-treatment for the "flare" is particularly important when a man has bone involvement. Spinal compression can occur during this period and adding the Casodex or Eulexin can reduce the risk of having this serious problem occur.

Following the failure of conventional hormonal treatment, low-dose DES, Premarin or PC-SPES (PC is for prostate cancer and SPES is the Latin word for hope) are sometimes used as secondary hormonal treatments. Years ago, high-dose DES was the mainstay of chemical hormonal treatment for advanced prostate cancer. When LH-RH became available, high-dose DES was no longer used, because it was causing heart attacks and blood clots and LH-RH treatment became available.

Interestingly, a friend of ours, Jim Charles, who is the President of the US-TOO support group in Houston, took a form of DES when his PSA began to rise after a radical prostatectomy and subsequent radiation. Since his rising PSA indicated treatment failure, Jim's next step was adjuvant radiation, which also failed. By then his PSA was rising one point every tens days, and not surprisingly, his fear factor was rising accordingly. At that point, he decided to try Honvan, a form of DES manufactured in Germany. His PSA returned to an undetectable status and has remained undetectable for over five years even though he stopped taking the Honvan a number of years ago. For reasons not understood, this also occurs sometimes with the LH-RH treatments. Although it is uncommon, Jim's case and that of others who have achieved remission after hormonal treatments are stopped, may provide scientists with important clues on why this complete remission of the cancer occurred.

Hank Porterfield, former chairman of US TOO, the largest network of prostate cancer support groups, learned about PC SPES supplements and initiated a study with a group of prostate cancer survivors. The promising data is not complete, but it clearly indicates an area for more research, some of which is now underway at several name-brand institutions.

Some men choose to have an **orchiectomy**, which is the surgical removal of the testes to deprive the cancer cells of male hormones. Because most testosterone is produced in the testicles, it is the surest and least expensive way to rid the body of the testosterone. In this outpatient procedure a small incision is made in the scrotum, and the testicles are removed. Since the scrotum is left intact with an orchiectomy, some men opt for reconstructive cosmetic surgery. A prosthesis similar in shape and size to the testes is placed in the scrotum.

An orchiectomy is also the quickest form of hormonal therapy. The testosterone from the testes plummets within hours of the surgery and disappears permanently. The downside of this therapy is its finality and the subsequent psychological effects of castration, especially now that intermittent hormonal therapy is being studied. This certainly stops the hormone production permanently, but it does not give room for a change of mind or a chance to restore normal sexual function should there be a cure for prostate cancer.

Both surgical and hormonal drug therapy produces drastic responses: the PSA decreases and the tumor and lymph nodes shrink. Hormonal deprivation is not considered to be curative and is seldom used as a primary treatment but is sometimes used before and after radiation and surgery. It is important to note that hormonal therapy is a major treatment for metastatic disease.

Chemotherapy

Chemotherapy involves the use of toxic compounds, most of which are derived from "mother nature," to kill cancer cells. In the past, chemotherapy was not considered to be very effective for prostate cancer, but recently this thinking is beginning to change, particularly in the area of palliative therapy. Palliative therapy is non-curative treatment to relieve a patient's symptoms and improve his quality of life. If a man responds to chemotherapy, he usually improves his overall health as well as minimizing the intensity and duration of his pain. Today, combinations of drugs are showing promise to extend life as well as improve the quality of life and even bring about a remission, but as yet, these drugs do not show evidence of achieving a cure.

Chemotherapy kills healthy as well as malignant cells, but the chemotherapy drugs currently used for prostate cancer are not as toxic as those used for other cancers, so the side effects are generally less severe. New drugs are being developed and tested in combination with existing drugs to obtain improved responses with fewer side effects. Trials are also underway to use chemotherapy at an earlier stage, even before conventional primary treatment.

One of the chemotherapies being studied is the combination of **Emcyt** and **Taxotere**. Emcyt (estramustine) is an estrogen related drug that has shown evidence of reducing testosterone while killing cancer cells. Unfortunately, the side effects are difficult. Since Emcyt is drug that is taken daily, the risk of heart attacks, nausea and blood clots are increased. By combining Emcyt with Taxotere and changing the dosage, scientists hope to achieve better results with fewer side effects.

Most of the present studies of combinations of chemotherapies have been able to improve the quality of life, but, until recently, they did not improve the survival rate. However, now there is not only great hope the survival rate will improve, there is scientific evidence that survival rates have already improved with chemotherapy.

Recently, I sat at an US TOO meeting in Houston with a large group of men and women, all of whom were eager to hear Dr. Christopher Logothetis tell us about his astounding work with chemotherapy and the promising results he and his colleagues were achieving.

He explained how his team was tailoring combinations of chemotherapies for individuals with advanced prostate cancer and in one study, they had achieved a high biochemical survival rate at four years after treatment. This was astonishing news. In the past, there was little evidence of the benefit of chemotherapy on survival. Now there has been a remarkable leap forward in just a few years, a leap that translates to real change and hope for patients now, not just those who will be patients in the distant future.

He also enlightened us on an upcoming research trial with **Gleevec** and **Taxotere**. Gleevec is the cancer killing chemotherapy that has been in the news lately. Dr. Logothetis and his team have already shown that by using this combination in mice with prostate cancer bone metastasis, they could rid the bone of cancer. Targeting cancer in the bone is very important as the pattern prostate cancer usually takes is to head for the bone, and 80% of men who die of prostate cancer have bone metastasis. Making bone hostile to cancer growth is an exciting project. Dr. Logothetis will head the research on the combination of Gleevec and Taxotere scheduled to begin shortly at MDACC.

The study participants are excited about this new development not only because they believe it will improve their lives, but also because they can work with Dr. Logothetis, who is one of the most admired and loved specialists in the cancer world.

Chemotherapy is also very important for small cell carcinoma of the prostate, which has the initial appearance of the common form of prostate cancer. After treatment, however, small cell carcinoma can return with a vengeance, rapidly growing in the prostate bed and spreading quickly to the bone, lungs, brain and liver. Amazingly, a man with this form of the disease may continue to have a low PSA as the cancer is aggressively spreading through his body. Generally, he is prescribed combinations of chemotherapies, including Platinol, Taxol, Taxotere, and several others. At times, radiation is also performed.

## Watchful Waiting

Prostate cancer is often described as a disease that men die "with" not "of." That is because, basically, 42% of men will develop cancer cells in the prostate during their lifetimes, but only 3% will die of the disease. For years, this slow growing natural history lulled the public into placing prostate cancer in the "not too dangerous" category. However, as the 31,500 prostate cancer deaths per year indicate, prostate cancer is potentially lethal.

As a result of the reputation for slow growth, after diagnosis, some men choose to watch the progression of their PSA before undertaking surgery, radiation or another treatment. This approach enables them to avoid, at least for a period of time, the complications from surgery or radiation and the attendant side effects.

"Watchful waiting" is generally used for men with a very low PSA who have very small, well-differentiated tumors. In this case, the expectation is that a long time will elapse before treatment is necessary. Others who choose this approach include elderly men with a life expectancy of less than ten years, or debilitated patients who are too ill for treatment.

The downside of this approach is that, since the cancer can actually be more aggressive or more widespread than it may appear at diagnosis, the man may end up forfeiting his chance to be cured. It is interesting to note that controversy and emotions are very strong concerning this issue in both the medical and patient community.

If "watchful waiting" is applicable in your partner's case, his physician will carefully monitor the growth of the tumor and the rate of change by repeating a PSA every six months or less or by performing another biopsy until the rate that the cancer is growing becomes clearer.

Even with this information, "watchful waiting" is still the most difficult choice to make regarding treatment. The tests that are presently available cannot predict whether or not a tumor will remain small and indolent. For example, one study reported that 25% of the participants with progressing tumors had PSA's that remained unchanged.

Nevertheless, some men are willing to live in this uncertain situation to delay the complications and side effects of treatment, but others are not willing to bear either the worry that the cancer is quietly growing and escaping the prostate or the concern that they missed a "window of opportunity."

## The Dilemma

Since the advent of the PSA and other improved diagnostic tools, men are receiving early rather than late stage diagnoses. They are then bewildered by the question of whether they can live a good bit longer without therapy or be cured if they initiate aggressive therapy. The decision facing them is especially difficult since they don't know if the radical approach will, indeed, secure a cure or if waiting will be too much of a risk for them to handle emotionally and physically.

A man's choice in this area is not made easier by the number of conflicting opinions and fierce debates about treatments even within the medical community, where experts reach different conclusions from the same evidence.

Also, it's a well-known fact that specialists are generally biased toward their own field. It makes sense that a surgeon would be more likely than a radiation oncologist to suggest a prostatectomy and vice versa. To me, it would seem that physicians in a certain specialty might impose treatment prejudices on their patients without even being aware that theirs is not the most objective view.

The patient's dilemma is compounded by the fact that just the word "cancer" can scare a man into a treatment that may not be appropriate for him. Education and understanding about each treatment option definitely improves the decision-making process.

Dick's example truly illustrates the basic quandary that most men face when they choose to watch and wait. In Dick's situation, his supposedly plain vanilla case was far more aggressive than the PSA or biopsy indicated. His post surgery pathology also showed the cancer was into and not through the wall of the prostate on both sides. Had he chosen the "watchful waiting" route, he might have given up his chance for a cure.

For him, in fact, "watchful waiting" was never an option. First, he rarely waits for any reason. Customarily, his tendency is to press forward even if forward is the wrong direction. In his case, pressing on with a radical prostatectomy was the correct direction and a decision that saved his life.

Dick continues to maintain that men should give greater consideration to the treatment that is most likely to cure the cancer as opposed to making the decision based primarily on treatment side effects.

Stated another way: if the treatment is not successful, the side effects become far less important. Although each man or each couple must make the decision they feel is right for them, both of us feel that men and women can work together to find solutions for the side effects of prostate cancer. In contrast, if the disease is metastatic to nodes or bone, it is not curable.

So if the man you love has a good chance for a cure, you might encourage him not to postpone treatment because of concern over side effects. Help him understand that you love him completely and that you will remain by his side as the two of you work on the side effects together. Although many men and women are not comfortable discussing these matters, the two of you might benefit by taking a different approach and openly expressing your thoughts on these matters.

## *Planning Ahead*

When Dick received his diagnosis, he found consolation in focusing on business matters and putting his "affairs in order." Although Dick's surgery date was set as early as possible, he still had time to redo his will, settle his financial affairs, prepare his obituary and detail his funeral arrangements. At the doctor's suggestion, he prepared for blood loss during the surgery by donating his own blood in advance. (This is a good suggestion for anyone who might need a transfusion, although today's blood-sparing techniques minimize the need for transfusion, and the quality of the blood in the blood banks has greatly improved.)

He even organized a "Black Book" that outlined everything Charlotte needed to know about their financial affairs, as well as how to dispose of their collections and other steps she should take in case of his death. His actions were loving, caring steps to secure Charlotte's future in case his prostate cancer was more severe than he thought.

His impressions were so skewed toward a less than promising future that he once told me, "During that period, I wouldn't even buy a new pair of shoes."

Focusing on these business transactions also provided much needed diversions for his anxious mind. I have noticed that Dick absorbs himself in a major project requiring either great mental concentration or physical strength when he is most upset. Every person has his or her own way of riding through a difficult emotional storm.

Mentioning Dick's actions is not meant to imply that such practical steps should be avoided. I merely wanted to point out that many men, even the strongest, are dealing with a huge emotional overload after their diagnosis and need an extra measure of a woman's love, understanding, respect and coping skills.

Helping to ease the man's load and being a special comforter and helpmate is a major role for the woman in his life. And that role is not simple, because when dealing with a crisis as potentially devastating as prostate cancer, she needs to be sensitive as to how best to help him cope emotionally and tend to the pragmatic matters of his life.

For example, once when my deceased husband, James, was very tired from both his cancer treatments and huge business problems, he looked at me and said, "I feel like throwing down my sword and quitting the fight." I knew that my words would be meaningless at that moment, so I said very little, gave him a hug and set about implementing what I feel was a divinely inspired plan to encourage him. As soon as James was occupied with another business call, I used our second line and called a number of antique shops until I found one that had an old sword in the inventory. I raced to the shop, brought the sword and brought it home in a big brown paper bag. It was not an elaborate or expensive piece, but it carried a very valuable message.

By the time I arrived, James was quietly sitting alone in his favorite chair in a dreadfully morose state. This was very unusual for him as he rarely complained and always maintained a hopeful, positive attitude. I handed him the oddly shaped dull brown package. When he pulled out the sword, he was overcome with emotion. I cannot explain the emotional healing that took place when he received that one small gift, but it was outwardly evident that his spirits had been lifted. I lovingly wiped the tears from his face and went about my work as usual, trying to give him an opportunity to assimilate his feelings.

On a practical level, his "sword" was the weapon he needed for the business fight ahead of him, too. He dove into his business crisis like General Patton and at the end of his busy day, he slammed his briefcase shut with a satisfied click, and we walked out our front door for a long happy walk in the moonlight.

Dick has had his "need-a-sword" moments as well, and I have used other diversionary measures for him, particularly when he awaits the results of each new PSA. He isn't always aware of his rising stress level during that period of time, but I can tell. Dick is a very good-natured person, so if he is the least bit testy, something is bothering him. I usually suggest that we head for the lake home for a few days, or I plan an evening with friends. Once I gathered candles from around our home, lit thirty of them in the bathroom and drew a hot bath for him. After his bath, I moved the candles to the bedroom, brought him dinner in bed and presented him with a good mystery novel. A doctor was the sleuth and main character, which I hoped would satisfy his medical bent.

Most of us, however, cannot be patient, thoughtful and creative all of the time. Unfortunately, if I am very tired and cranky, I don't interact with Dick as patiently as I should either. These times remind me of the importance of rest when things are distressing. I can't raise my own sword when I am too tired to retrieve it from its scabbard.

Dick also has his own array of defensive and offensive "swords" for the many men who call him for information about prostate cancer. It is not unusual for him to stop during a conversation and make mention of a particular medical article that details a specific treatment that might be helpful to the caller. As soon as he finishes his visit with the prostate cancer survivor, he quickly copies the articles he has in mind for the man's specific circumstances and mails them that day. He has told me many times how important it is to get life-saving and hope-saving data in the hands of survivors as quickly as possible. In short, his "swords" are weapons that open up a world of light and as they hope cut away the darkness that is ever-present when a person lacks knowledge about his own health.

Although he accomplished all the business matters at hand prior to entering the hospital, what Dick didn't do was tell his three sons about his diagnosis until the night before his surgery. At that point, he called each one individually and shared the news about his prostate cancer diagnosis and his radical prostatectomy, which was scheduled for the following morning. Since cancer is a family disease, he now admits that this was not a good strategy. Family members need the opportunity to support and console one another. In trying to protect his sons, he unknowingly robbed them of the opportunity to lend their assistance. Dick also made the mistake of not sharing his situation with his closest friends. Close friends want to support one another when life has taken a foul turn.

## The Surgery

Dick and Charlotte remained apprehensive and rarely communicated with each other about the upcoming surgery. It is interesting that some people deal quietly with their anxiety and others need to articulate their fears. James and I were "in the head and out the mouth" personalities, so we lived with few unexpressed thoughts. The important point is for each of you to cope in the way you find most comfortable, without leaving one of the partners feeling distant from the other. Fortunately, Dick and Charlotte's heavy-heartedness improved over time, and by the surgery date, they replaced their apprehension with hopefulness and more conversation.

Upon arrival at the hospital, Dick filled out the usual hospital consent forms and had the usual blood tests. After he settled into his hospital bed, he was interrupted repeatedly by a number of different doctors. Each one examined him and then performed his own version of the "dreaded rectal examination" (DRE). After enduring repeated DRE's from all of the different doctors, Dick thought surgery was beginning to look like a piece of cake.

The surgery the following morning went well but lasted five rather than the anticipated three hours. When he woke up in the recovery room, Dick became agitated when none of the nurses would tell him if his prostate had been removed. He knew that if biopsies of his lymph nodes were positive, the surgeon would not remove the prostate, and his prognosis would be bleak.

Only after he was finally taken back to his hospital room did he hear the good news that his prostate was removed, and the laboratory analysis of his lymph nodes was negative. Thrilled with this information, Dick inspected his incision, which ran from the navel to the penis, the avenue of the retropubic radical prostatectomy, as opposed to the perineal approach with the incision between the anus and the scrotum.

During surgery, a Foley catheter is inserted into the penis and is anchored by a small balloon in the bladder. Now Dick tells others who are awaiting surgery, to reach down and feel if they have a catheter taped to their leg after they awake in the recovery room. Generally, if they have a catheter, they can know right away that their prostate has been removed. This is not necessarily the case, but it happens more often than not and is a comforting sign in the recovery room where information is limited.

Early on the first day after the surgery, Dick was allowed to eat what he wanted as long as it was not constipating, and he was encouraged to walk. The nurse placed the urine bag in full view on his rolling pole along with the IV fluids and the automatic pump for the pain medications in preparation for the walk.

Walking was important to improve his circulation, reduce the risk of blood clots and also to awaken his bowels. Constipation can occur easily from the pain medications, dehydration and inactivity. Since the rectum is very fragile for several months after surgery, it is important to have a bowel movement every day. Otherwise the rectum could become injured from straining with constipation. In fact, he was also told not to do any activity, like taking an enema that could perforate his rectum. So to keep things moving, Dick took his stool softeners and reluctantly followed his instructions to walk the hospital halls.

The second day he "hit the pain wall," which seems to be normal fare for many surgical patients. Normal or not, every minute of real time seemed like an hour to him and every hour felt like a century, but the pain eventually subsided to a manageable state by the third day. Also on the third day, the doctor arrived to remove the two suction drains that had been placed in his abdomen to drain fluid from the area where the prostate was removed. The doctor told Dick that the procedure was not painful and that he would only feel a little pressure. However, when the doctor cut the sutures and pulled out the drains, Dick likened the experience to having his intestines pulled through a small hole in his abdomen, a sentiment shared by many prostate cancer survivors. Fortunately, after the drains were removed, he improved quickly and was released three days later, a long stay compared to the current two to three day stays after a radical prostatectomy.

Before his release, the doctor removed the surgical staples that held the incision together and replaced them with "steri-strips," which stayed on for about a week until his body began healing itself. Fortunately, he was able to take a shower by covering the strips with plastic wrap. Along with his list of medication instructions, he was told to avoid lifting and strenuous activity. For a man whose hobby is major construction work, this was bad news.

The good news was that the cancer was no longer in his body but in a pathology lab. As it turned out, with Gleason scores and staging in mind, the pathology performed after Dick's prostate was removed told a somewhat different story than the original biopsy. He actually had a Gleason 3+4=7, which indicates a significantly more aggressive tumor than a 3+3=6. Also, the cancer extended into but not through the capsule of the prostate and was in both sides of the prostate. His stage was now a T2c-N-Zero-M Zero. In other words, he had a very close call. As Dick often says, "Thank God for the PSA test!"

## *Home Again*

Dick and Charlotte returned home from the hospital with high hopes and his handy Foley catheter still in place. He was given a prescription for antibiotics to minimize the risk of infection, which he was to begin taking before the catheter is removed. The catheter was left in the penis temporarily to allow the site where the urethra and the bladder were connected time to heal. Dick was told to be careful with the catheter and to keep it taped securely to his thigh, because if he inadvertently pulled it out, he could do such damage that he would be permanently incontinent or, at least, require surgery to reinstall it.

He was also given a "don't worry if this happens" list by his doctor. Be sure to ask for such a list so you will not be overly concerned if you see some blood in the urine bag or a number of other startling but innocuous happenings.

The day after he left the hospital, he and Charlotte drove to their lake home three hours from Houston and then on to New Orleans, where Dick gave two forty-five minute presentations to a group of mechanical musical instrument collectors. With the catheter bag strapped to his leg, Dick enthusiastically expounded about player pianos and nickelodeons to the collectors on hand. In looking back, he believes he would have had a more favorable recovery if he had not undertaken such a heavy post surgery travel and activity schedule. The catheter worked well enough for him to carry on with his regular life, and he feels he should have been satisfied with just that during his recovery period.

## *Post-surgical Incontinence*

Usually, after the initial treatment of prostate cancer, men experience some degree of incontinence. Most men generally improve within a year and can even achieve total continence, but it can be a slow process. Certain exercises (see page 99) have proven to help strengthen the sphincter muscles and improve urinary control. In addition, there are a number of products with varying degrees of absorbency, which are helpful until the man achieves complete urinary control, such as pads and washable underwear with built in absorbency. The problem with the underwear is that it is not a good product for travel outside of the country, as it requires a long time to dry when laundry service is not handy.

Urinary incontinence from surgery occurs when one or both sphincters are damaged or destroyed. The internal urethral sphincter, which is located in the bladder neck, provides involuntary urine control. The damage occurs when the urethra is severed at the base of the bladder, which destroys the internal (upper) sphincter. The external (lower) sphincter may be traumatized during the radical prostatectomy. Most men have significant incontinence when the catheter is removed until the external sphincter heals and recovers enough to be retrained, however, the extent of the urinary control that remains after a few weeks or months varies widely from complete control to some incontinence to total incontinence. Fortunately, complete incontinence is uncommon.

New surgical techniques to reduce the risk of incontinence are being developed. Some surgical steps that are being tried to help preserve continence are techniques to reconnect the bladder and the urethra, better placement of the urethral sutures and avoidance of traction on the urethra during surgery.

After surgery, scar tissue can occur and cause a urethral stricture or bladder neck contracture. That is why it is important to report urine flow reductions to the urologist, who can correct the problem with a simple procedure.

There are a number of minimally invasive therapies that can help stress incontinence. Various types of electrical stimulation, electromagnetic fields and biofeedback have been touted as useful.  Some men have used small electrical shocks to stimulate and build up the sphincter muscles, which they tout sometimes improves their continence. This electrical stimulation is basically painless and can be administered in a doctor's office or with a battery powered implant.

Stopping urine flow midstream (see below) has helped some men considerably by strengthening the pelvic muscles and the muscles of the external sphincter, which, in turn, enhances urine control. There are some medications that can be used for post-prostatectomy incontinence but their efficacy is so low that many urologists don't even prescribe them.

As for questions regarding the affect of cranberry juice, cranberry pills and caffeine, it is my understanding that cranberry juice helps acidify urine, which, in turn, decreases the incidence of infection. The correlation is that these cranberry products may, in turn, reduce the incidence of incontinence related to urinary tract infections. Caffeine is another matter. It is a diuretic, which causes the bladder to fill and can irritate the bladder, so for these reasons, limiting caffeine may reduce incontinence.

My favorite name for a non-invasive product is the "Geezer Squeezer," which is a clamp for controlling incontinence. I have heard that this control device helps stop leakage more comfortably than other clamping devices, because it puts pressure on the urethra in the lower part of the penis and avoids pressure on the top of the penis where there are more nerves.

Since these non-invasive therapies are relatively new, long-range data on their effectiveness or side effects is not established. The main issue is to know that there are solutions for incontinence and special products to help the situation while you are seeking the correct solution.

Like most men, Dick's problem with incontinence started when the catheter was removed in his urologist's office two weeks following surgery. Although the nurse had told him to bring a pad for his underwear, she neglected to mention what type of pad to bring, so he purchased a package of mini-pads. He inserted the thin pad into his underwear and headed for the car with Charlotte. To their surprise, by the time they reached the car, Dick's trousers were soaked and his shoes were filled with urine. This was his welcome to the world of urinary incontinence!

He immediately purchased a pack of **extra absorbency pads** at his neighborhood drug store. Although they worked fairly well, the moisture caused him to have a severe rash. To combat the rash, he invented an external catheter, which could be attached to a bag to hold urine. Later, he discovered that this device was already available as a condom catheter at medical supply stores. He wanted to send one to his congressman to use when participating in filibusters, because with these catheters and a few leg bags, there would be no need to leave the podium for days.

When the **condom catheters** also caused a rash, Dick recognized that he had a very serious problem. Ever the engineer, he next invented what he called the "Dick in the Bag." It was a one-gallon plastic bag tied around his waist with a hole punched in it to collect the urine. All was well until he was attending a dinner party one evening and forgot about the new invention. Suddenly, the bag was about ready to burst, so he beat a hasty retreat to the bathroom, emptied the bag, reinstalled it and returned to the table with a huge sigh of relief. He still worries about what would have happened if two quarts of his urine had suddenly ended up on the terrazzo floor under the dinner table.

Sadly, such incidents have happened to other men. Knowing what to expect helps prevent these episodes. This story serves as another example to illustrate that when men speak openly with one another about their own experience, they acquire a wealth of knowledge not just about the medical aspects of cancer but also tips on making every day life easier after undertaking cancer treatment.

For example, we recently learned that Dr Walsh suggests that men can improve their continence more quickly if they do not wear a condom catheter, an attached bag or clamp of any kind. By refraining from using one of these devices, they use their own muscles more readily and can regain their muscle control and urinary control quicker.

Another suggestion he has to help regain continence after surgery is to practice stopping the urine flow in mid-stream, which is done by tensing the muscles in the pelvic floor. However, it is important to take care not to overwork the sphincter by doing it too often.

After his dinner party experience, Dick started looking for another solution. He had heard stories about the early Texas cowboys with BPH, benign prostatic hyperplasia, a condition in which there is an overgrowth of prostate tissue that constricts the urethra and can block urine flow. To urinate, the cowboys used slender steel tubes to catheterize themselves out on the long trail rides. They would pull the makeshift catheters out of their hats, insert them and when finished, they would wipe off the tube between their thumb and forefinger and coil the tube back into their cowboy hats, remount their horses and head out onto the prairie to rope another cow. Dick dragged out his ten-gallon cowboy hat and plastic catheter, but fortunately, before he took such a drastic measure, the rash subsided. By then, he was able to return to using extra-absorbency pads, then regular-absorbency and on to special underwear with some built in absorbency and shaped pads called "Guards" for slight leakage.

But even the underwear became a hassle, so the search for a solution to his moderate incontinence continued. Soon thereafter, he became aware that **collagen injections** were being tested in clinical trials as bulking agents to control mild to moderate incontinence. Dick was given a skin test to make sure he was not allergic to the collagen and after the results proved negative, he became one of the first patients to receive these injections following FDA approval. The first injection worked well for about seven days, which was about the amount of time it took for the swelling to go down. Then the incontinence returned. The same was true for the second and third injections over a twelve-month period, but he forged ahead anyway.

The fourth injection greatly reduced the problem. This major triumph only lasted fifteen months, because collagen is eventually absorbed in the body.

Unfortunately, this procedure is extremely painful. It involves inserting a cystoscope, which is tube with a tiny television camera and a light source, into the penis and through the urethra to a point just above the sphincter. Then the collagen is injected. The procedure is performed in a doctor's office with only pain deadening salve for pain relief. Dick had a choice between this method and general anesthesia. Not wanting to place himself repeatedly under general anesthesia when it was not necessary, he chose the far more painful but less dangerous route.

By the time he had his eleventh injection, we were married, so I felt comfortable in accompanying him into the mini-operating room. I stood close to him and held his hand as I watched the doctor perform the procedure on the television screen. In my previous role as his driver on collagen injection days, I remained in the waiting room until the "operation" was complete. I was never comfortable with his metallic pallor or his obviously weakened state after each treatment, but I didn't say much, because he never complained except to say, "It smarts!"

After observing the procedure, I realized that "It smarts!" was a major understatement. At that point, I began to wage a major "nag" campaign. In my opinion, I felt he should not have the collagen injections again. Having encountered so very much pain with porphyria, the illness that has plagued me for decades, I am particularly sensitive to anyone who is suffering. I realize that pain cannot be the measure of whether a person should endure a specific medical procedure, but when the gain is questionable, it is time to readdress the issue. Dick, who is stoic in painful situations, even agreed that the pain was no longer relative to the gain.

So his search for a solution to control his mild incontinence problem began again. He learned about a new **male sling** for mild to moderate incontinence, which is manufactured by American Medical Systems (AMS). The male sling looks like a little hammock and is a modification of the female sling, which has been quite successful in treating stress incontinence in women for many years. It has only recently been available for use in men, so there is no long-term data available, but it looks quite promising.

Implanting the sling is a simple operation and takes only 45 minutes and provides the same bulking action as collagen. Three self-tapping screws are driven into both sides of the pubic bone to anchor the sling, which is generally made of an inert cadaveric material. It compresses the urethra against the pubic bone and thereby restricts urine flow.

Incontinence can be a very traumatic problem. Men, who are totally incontinent, are usually virtual prisoners of their incontinence until they solve the problem. Most tend to stay at home and stay horizontal, whenever possible. If they venture out, they usually wear dark trousers. Moreover, they also not only have to carry a supply of pads, they have to find places to change and dispose of them. Using twenty pads a day is certainly not uncommon. Just think of going on a five-day trip and having to deal with 100 pads!!

In fact, in the course of his business, an acquaintance of ours had to make many trips to the orient. He had to stop in several small, beautiful out of the way islands and a few large cities in Japan. What sounded like a three-week vacation was actually a three-week nightmare for him. He was totally incontinent and had to bring multiple suitcases full of heavy-duty pads leaving him little room for clothes. None of the vacation spots sold such pads, and if they did, there would hardly be enough on the island to meet his needs. As if that weren't enough of a problem, he added the frantic fear that he would have an accident during his important business meetings in Japan. Even though he was well padded, the pads sometimes leaked and ruined his clothes. So on the hottest of summer days, he had to wear dark slacks to hide any accidents.

Even such severe incontinence problems can usually be solved with an **artificial sphincter**. It is the most invasive treatment for incontinence, requiring hospitalization and anesthesia. This device consists of three elements: the cuff, the control pump and the pressure-regulating balloon. During surgery, a soft, stretchy cuff is fixed around the patient's urethra below the external sphincter. The pump is installed in the scrotum, and the balloon, which acts as a reservoir and is filled with a saline solution, is placed in the abdomen.

The cuff is normally closed and holds the urine in the bladder. When the man feels the urge to urinate, he reaches down and squeezes the pump about ten times. This opens the cuff by pumping the fluid back into the balloon. The urine then flows naturally out through the penis. After about two to three minutes, the fluid automatically returns from the balloon to the cuff to close it, in order to contain the next batch of urine. A double cuff version is also available for more difficult cases.

In the past, post-surgical infections and malfunction of the artificial sphincters were not uncommon. However, these new artificial sphincters are high tech devices with very high mechanical reliability and patient satisfaction. Like any mechanical device, they can have mechanical problems, but the satisfaction rate has been reported as 90% or higher. They are a Godsend to men who are totally incontinent and have no other options.

If your partner has a need for either of these devices or procedures, his urologist can provide information about their reliability and results.

After hearing Dick's matter of fact description of such a delicate subject, I wasn't bothered. I was beginning to be menopausal and knew that incontinence could easily happen to me. But more importantly, like most people who lose their spouses, I was focused on what is valuable in life. Continence was way down the list of the characteristics I sought in a man. Integrity, compassion, intelligence, humor, courage etc. were Dick's qualities, all of which were high on my check-list. It didn't hurt that he was very good looking, too. Solutions for incontinence were available, but cures for poor character are more difficult, if not impossible to find.

This does not negate the emotional upheaval that incontinence causes for men and their partners. Nevertheless, I firmly believe that a beautiful intimacy and healing partnership can develop in spite of such problems.

## Re-establishing Potency

Since marriage was probably going to be in our future, we agreed to have some in-depth conversations of a sexual nature, too. Before our conversation, I decided to read about the impotence problems related to the treatments for prostate cancer. I learned first that most men who are diagnosed with prostate cancer are middle-aged to older and are already confronting changes in their vitality and are extremely disturbed by their lowering hormone level and the subsequent decline of their potency. In other words, among other age-related problems, men may already be dealing with impotency problems of varying degrees, none of which are related to prostate cancer.

To illustrate this point, a 1994 New England Research Institute study reported that over half of the American men over forty had some measure of impotence, varying between minimal, moderate and total. The physical causes aside from those related to prostate cancer may include: alcohol, fatigue, vascular problems, particular drugs, illnesses or injuries that affect the spinal cord, endocrine system, pelvis, groin or those that cause severe pain or great stress. In addition, many men are facing retirement or are already retired and are adjusting to their new state of life, which can also cause stress that may affect a man's libido.

I was not surprised when I read about a study that showed that some men exaggerated their sexual prowess before treatment for prostate cancer. In the same study, men thought they were not potent after surgery and their wives thought they were. Unless there has been a follow-up study to explain the discrepancy, the incongruity is not clear. I have my own thoughts, which are not based on any science. I think it is related again to the general feeling of virility that decreases with age and anything that affects a man's feeling of virility affects a man's potency.

Researchers are also studying what they believe to be male menopause, which has been aptly named "viropause." Men experiencing "viropause" have a decline in strength, muscle mass and muscle tone. However, the physical symptoms of "viropause" are milder than as those found in female menopause. Apparently, however, the emotional strain of "viropause" is comparable to that of female menopause, causing such symptoms as depression, anxiety and fear. When a man faces aging issues and then adds the strain of prostate cancer, which could further drastically affect his manhood, he often becomes more vulnerable and more silent about his health and emotional problems than ever.

Dick and I gingerly broached the sexuality subject. Dick talked about impotence with the same pragmatic approach as if he were explaining the details of operating a drilling rig. He explained that impotence affected his ability to maintain an erection sufficient for intercourse, but it did not mean that he had lost his sexual drive, sensation or ability to have an orgasm.

After he recounted all the many methods he had used to try to reestablish his former potency, I was teary. He and so many other men have shown admirable courage in facing this traumatic dilemma with such confident attitudes. In Dick's case, he pressed forward to find a solution in spite of repeated failures. I was all the more admiring of this incredibly fine man, and regardless of his predicament, I felt that together we could find a way to change his circumstances.

Dick and his late wife Charlotte had tried most of the available methods to help with his impotence problem except for the non-prescription pills. Although these pills were heavily advertised, he looked on them as what we used to call "patent medicines." He told me, "I didn't try them, but I was tempted, because they had names like: Erogenex, Intimex, Testerex, Maximus and Top Gun!"

He continued our conversation by explaining that during his six-month check-up visit with the urologist following surgery, he told the doctor that he was still impotent. The doctor tried to be encouraging and said that sometimes it takes a year or more for a man to regain spontaneous potency after radical surgery. In the meantime, he suggested that Dick try a **vacuum tube device**, as it was the easiest, non-invasive, non-surgical procedure to achieve an erection.

Dick and Medicare spent $400 for the battery-powered apparatus, which Bill Martin aptly described in his book, *My Prostate and Me*, as a device that looks somewhat like a salad shooter. The principle of the device is to use a vacuum tube and pump to draw blood into the penis and retain the blood with a rubber band or constricting ring placed at the base of the penis. Then the vacuum tube is removed and the banded erection remains.

Dick tried it out in private and was disappointed with the results. The bottom line is that it he found the appliance awkward to use and quite painful when he snapped the rubber bands into place. Ouch! Sadly, he returned the device to its fancy bag and placed it on the top shelf of his closet.

Some men and women are very satisfied with the vacuum device. They are able to work through the strange, awkward stage and become proficient with it. Because of the band and the constriction, however, it is very important to make sure that the man consults with his doctor before using the appliance, principally if he has a physical ailment, such as a clotting problem.

Discouraged with the vacuum device and his continued state of impotence, he and Charlotte waited a very long year to seek other solutions. When Dick was ready to move forward, he visited Dr. Irving Fishman, a leading urologist in Houston who specializes in impotence. First, Dr. Fishman ran a Color Duplex Doppler test and determined that Dick had a venous leak, because the blood would return to the bloodstream before intercourse could be completed. Having a venous leak made it unlikely that Dick could ever sustain an erection on his own again. After this disheartening news, the doctor suggested that he try the **tri-mix shots**, a mixture of papavarine, prostaglandin and phentolamine, which are injected directly into the penis. While these shots produced a satisfactory erection in about five minutes, it was necessary for Dick to use the highest dosage in order to overcome the venous leak.

Using such a high dose concerned him, because he was beginning to experience residual pain.

When Dick learned that there was a clinical trial underway using **MUSE** (Medicated Urethral Suppository for Erection), he decided to try it. MUSE is a suppository about the size of a pencil lead, which is composed of one of the same drugs found in the shots. It is placed in the penis with a short wand and creates an erection in ten to fifteen minutes. The first administration of MUSE should be performed under medical supervision. The man should urinate prior to inserting the pellet. The small amount of urine left in the urethra is enough to lubricate the urinary tract for easier application of the MUSE. Other lubricants like Vasoline can interfere with the absorption of the drug. The penis should be pulled upward and outward to straighten the urethra before inserting the wand. This helps minimize or prevent pain for most men.

Dick quickly enrolled in the trial with the thought that a suppository sounded much better than shots. As part of the protocol, he returned to his doctor's office each week, where he received the treatment dose and was then measured before and after the MUSE to determine the results of various doses.

MUSE didn't work well for Dick except on one favorable occasion. To celebrate the moment, Dick spotted a "smiley face" ☺ sticker on the nurse's desk and applied it on the tip of his erection, where the nurse could not miss the happy results. When she pulled back the sheet to take her required research measurements, she howled with laughter when she saw the ☺ grinning up at her. With the exception of this solitary successful treatment, MUSE did not work for him even at the highest dose. Nevertheless, MUSE has worked very well for many other men. I do not want to give the impression that Dick's experience is common to all.

Eventually, Dick returned to the shots, but the residual pain from the shots finally became unbearable. He also became concerned that he could develop a penile curvature problem similar to **Peyronie's disease**. With this condition, the penis develops plaque or scarring, which results in a curvature of the penis. The cause is not known, but tri-mix shots are thought by some to cause or aggravate penile curvature. There is still no definitive treatment but some physicians are trying verapamil hydrochloride, a topical drug, or therapy with a high dose Vitamin E and colchicine. Penile curvature can be corrected surgically, but it is a difficult undertaking.

Another problem sometimes seen with the tri-mix shots is **priapism**, a painful persistent erection that can last hours or even days. Although some men have joked that this is their ultimate fantasy, it is a serious condition, which can lead to irreversible impotence if it is not treated properly. Therefore, if this condition persists for four hours, a trip to the emergency room to have it chemically reversed is mandatory. Although Dick never had a priapism, the intense pain he was experiencing when he used the shots, coupled with these other issues, resulted in Dick's decision to discontinue them and begin contemplating what to do next.

During those days, **Viagra** had not been approved and was, therefore, not available to the public. At a later date, Dick did try the new blockbuster drug but with little success.

Viagra facilitates blood flow in the penis by relaxing the arteries in the penis through a complex mechanism, at which point an erection can occur. Viagra does not create an immediate erection but takes about an hour to come to full strength. There are a few suggestions to help facilitate the absorption of the drug. Enjoying a hot bath is one, because it increases blood flow to the penis, but primarily, Viagra requires tactile sexual stimulation.

Unfortunately, Dick's venous leak from his radical prostatectomy virtually eliminated the effect of the Viagra. Another unfortunate problem was that he was one of the men taking Viagra who had unusual symptoms like having a bluish tint in his vision. Fearful that if he gave the pills to another man, the recipient could develop this same problem or worse, Dick flushed all of his pills down the toilet. Considering that the 60 pills cost approximately $10 each, this was a $600 royal flush.

If your partner has any of the following medical conditions, Viagra is not recommended:

- Irregular heartbeat or recent heart attack
- Congestive heart failure
- Chest pain
- Blood pressure lower than 90/50
- Blood pressure higher than 170/110
- Retinitis pigmentosa
- History of cardiovascular disease
- Nitroglycerin or nitrate prescriptions

At this writing, however, eight million men have used Viagra and 75% of them are satisfied with the results; an excellent satisfaction rate. Shortly after Viagra was released, I found out that it was working extremely well.

Early one Saturday morning, I headed to my nearby drugstore to get some insulin. I was surprised to see a long line of men in front of the pharmacy window. I watched as the first gentleman handed in his prescription and waited patiently until it was filled. One man near the front of the line started conversing with the men around him about his treasured Viagra prescription, and soon the other nine men realized they were waiting for the same thing. While they laughed about their upcoming Saturday night, I blushed!

The advent of Viagra has also spurred men to seek sexual counseling and physical help. One study conducted by Pfizer, the manufacturer of Viagra, indicated that 15% sought counseling after Viagra became available as opposed to 7% beforehand.

A number of surgeons are now recommending that Viagra be used earlier rather than later after surgery. Some even prescribe it shortly after the patient leaves the hospital, not for intercourse but to "wake up" the nerves. If the nerve sparing procedure is not successful, Viagra will not work, but, fortunately, the tri-mix shots will. The future data on the use of Viagra pre-and post-surgery should prove very interesting.

*The Ultimate Solution for Impotence*

Unfortunately, Dick's beloved wife, Charlotte, died of a heart attack about the time they decided to stop using the shots. Saddened by her death, he placed the dilemma of his impotency and his search for a solution along with many other problems on the back burner of his life. Being a widower was tragic. Being an impotent and incontinent widower was an added anguish when he thought of the future without her love, her presence, her comfort and her understanding. He sorely missed the woman who had been his closest friend and who had been by his side since they were college students. Finding someone else with whom he could share such camaraderie would be difficult. Finding a woman with whom he could deal with his side effects from prostate cancer with the ease he had with Charlotte would be a complex undertaking. He discovered the depth of the problem on his first outing as a widower.

In the course of conversation with his first dinner partner, he mentioned prostate cancer. Surprisingly, she cautioned him saying that she thought it was best that he avoid this subject with women. He told me later, "I knew then that finding a woman who was supportive and communicative about prostate cancer was going to be difficult but essential to my future well being."

Dick's timing in revealing such personal information was, perhaps, a bit hasty, but it is interesting to see how single people deal with cancer when they are revealing the news to the opposite sex. Some people quickly divulge information about their cancer to potential partners in order to find out quickly if that person is going to reject them because of the cancer or if the person is hesitant to develop a relationship with someone with cancer.

Others promptly reveal details of their cancer, because they want to set themselves apart from the "victim" category, preferring to be perceived as strong, productive people.

Doesn't the Good Book say that the truth will set us free? Communication is freeing, but it is important to let people communicate about their illness at their own tempo whether it means telling the world immediately or refraining from talking about the diagnosis until the person is ready. Where sexual matters are concerned, using basic good manners is an excellent guidelines.

The same responses hold true for married couples, including the fear of rejection. In her book, *Sexuality and Fertility After Cancer*, Dr. Leslie Schover notes that it is more common for men to reject women after a cancer diagnosis than the reverse. She further contends that this may be due to the fact that women are accustomed to the idea of taking care of their mates, particularly if they marry someone older. As noted before, most women are experienced at being the caretakers for their children, family and friends.

Mostly, cancer survivors tell their new friend the details of their health history, because they are by nature open and forthright. Maybe, this was why Dick told me he was a prostate cancer survivor soon after we met. My reaction must have been his litmus test. Apparently I passed. I do think, however, it is better to develop a keen friendship before divulging details about your health.

Although I was eager to hear more about his case in our early courting days, I wasn't quite ready for the topic he decided to broach. Dick told me that he was impotent and that the only option he had left for a normal sexual life was to have a penile implant. Since he had already spent many years chasing the wrong solutions, he wanted to take action right away, particularly in light of our recent marriage discussions. I shuddered when he alerted me about his decision to have the operation.

I wanted to talk about the emotional implications of this surgery. Dick wanted to limit our discussions to matter of fact data about the device, including showing me a photograph and a diagram illustrating how it operates. When I saw the three-piece model of the implant device, my reaction was worse than when we were merely talking about it. The whole idea did not appeal to me, but Dick appealed to me, so I had to at least address the issue and help him through the surgery.

He investigated the three basic types of penile implant devices available, all of which do not disturb the natural look or feel of the penis. The simplest is the **semi-rigid device**, which is a rod or a pair of rods implanted in the penis, which can then be can be bent upward for intercourse and downward afterward. This device is easy to use and easier to install than the inflatable devices. The obvious disadvantage is that the penis is never flaccid. It is either bowed up or down.

Another option is the more complex, **self-contained inflatable implant**. It consists of two fluid filled cylinders, which are implanted in the penis, and a pump mechanism that is implanted beneath the glans or head of the penis. The device can be inflated by squeezing the head of the penis and deflated by bending the penis at the glans. Although this mechanism is simple, it is, nonetheless, more difficult to operate than the semi-rigid device.

The **three-piece penile implant** consists of three elements: the pump, two cylinders and a reservoir. The pump is installed in the scrotum for easy accessibility. The cylinders are inserted in the corpus cavernosa in the penis, and the reservoir, which is filled with a saline mixture, is placed in the abdomen. The tubes are fitted to the patient in the operating room by using different sizes, sleeves, and/or extension tips.

To get an erection, the man squeezes the pump to inflate the cylinders with fluid from the reservoir. In the 700 CX, the cylinders expand in girth but not in length. In another model, they expand in both girth and length. At the completion of intercourse, the man presses the deflation site on the pump, and the fluid flows back into the reservoir. The inflation process is quick, and a man's appearance in the locker room is very natural.

After scrutinizing the different types of devices, Dick chose the "gold standard" 700 CX, a fully inflatable device made by American Medical Systems. It was also the one most highly recommended by his surgeon, Dr Fishman. We have since learned that American Medical Systems has an excellent patient information service. Patients can call an 800 number (see page 172) and speak with the AMS patient liaison, who is available to answer their questions about the various devices. The company has also improved the 700 CX since Dick had his implanted by adding a Parylene coating to enhance its durability and an antibiotic coating to reduce the risk of infection.

Before he took such a final step, he spoke with men who had the implant surgery and asked their opinion. All of them seemed happy with the results, which was in line with the 90% satisfaction rate in a number of studies Dick had read. Confident that his choice was the best, he was ready to proceed with the penile implant surgery and once again become a paramour, thanks to a bionic part.

I was satisfied that he was in good medical hands. Dr. Fishman, who had helped Dick along the journey to potency, would be the surgeon. He was renowned in the field and had done many of these procedures. Dick asked me to come with him to several of his pre-op appointments with Dr. Fishman. Since we weren't married yet, I was taken aback and embarrassed both by the subject of the visit with Dr. Fishman and my role after the surgery. However, Dick needed someone to care for him once he got home from the hospital, so I decided that I should learn about his post-surgical medical requirements and be aware of what to do in case of an emergency. Fortunately, the nursing requirements were more in the line of bringing food and pills rather than bandages or some other treatment of the organ in question, so I willingly agreed to take the job.

When the day of the surgery arrived, I was there to hold his hand and act as a consoling companion during his short hospital stay. As you can imagine, I was not my usual chatty self with our friends when they asked why Dick was being admitted to the hospital for a few days. Instead of giving them explicit details, I tempered my conversations with, "It's a prostate cancer related problem, but don't worry. The cancer has not returned." My brief reply seemed to satisfy most people. Friends don't usually probe when something involves certain regions of the body, particularly the middle third.

After Dick was released from the hospital, I returned to Dick's house with him while he recovered. After you read my version of the recovery period, you will understand why. You will also see clearly why it is important to get a female's perspective on health situations.

The following is Dick's version of the surgery and the outcome:

"The surgery lasted a little more than an hour and was not difficult. My hospital stay was only a few days, and my recovery time at home was short as well: about two weeks to recover fully. The important thing is that, after waiting the mandatory total of five weeks before using the new implant, the device worked perfectly.

"Although I thought it would be difficult to locate the pump in my scrotum, it was easy. After approximately 30 pump strokes and a few minutes of time, I had an erection. It was simple to use, involved no pain, and took little time to activate. Most importantly, it functioned exactly like the natural erections that I had enjoyed in years past. What more can I say!"

My account of his surgery and recovery differs somewhat.

Although most men have an easy time with this particular surgery, Dick did not. He was in great pain in the hospital and despite my admonition to remain there, he insisted that was feeling much improved and checked out of the hospital far too soon. I do not blame Dr. Fishman, because Dick answered all of his "How are you feeling?" with the "I'm fine!" gusto of a man ready to get out of the hospital as fast as possible.

This happens frequently with patients of both genders but especially with males. Also, what I call the "98.6 factor" came into play during his interchanges with the doctor. As soon as people are in the presence of a doctor, they feel better and their temperature drops. How many times have mothers rushed their crying baby to the doctor's office with a temperature of 104. Then when the doctor walks in the examining room with the baby, the temperature slides down the thermometer from 104 to a normal 98.6.

Dick's situation was similar. He was very ill, weak and in pain. As soon as Dr. Fishman walked in the room, Dick felt a bit better and told Dr. Fishman that he was doing well and could go home. Having taken care of so many sick people and having been in the same situation myself, I have seen and experienced this behavior often. Although it feels emotionally better to hold back complaints, it does not help the doctor diagnosis your problem. Since Dick was more interested in maintaining his status as a non-complainer rather than being truthful about his pain and weakness, he gave Dr Fishman the wrong information. I was a better judge of his condition and was convinced he should remain in the hospital. We found out that I was right as soon as he was home, when he had to immediately return to the hospital and spend half of the night in the emergency room.

The next month was very difficult for him. He remained sick, weak and needed a great deal of care. I was the caregiver, so what could have been a short hospital stay with help from many nurses, was a month of night and day responsibility for me and sadly, continued illness for Dick.

I share this account not to grumble about caring for Dick, but to encourage caregivers to hold tight to their convictions and instincts. I could have saved Dick a great deal of agony and illness and me a month of a different kind of hardship had I only insisted that he remain in the hospital until we discovered what was causing him to be so ill. If that didn't work, I should have spoken with his nurse and his doctor.

Later we discovered that his condition was not related to the surgical procedure but rather to his previously unknown drug allergies. That problem could have been far more quickly resolved in the hospital than at home. The subsequent trips to the emergency room and the doctors office were difficult for someone as sick as Dick. He continued to have allergic reactions to the pain medications, which in turn, made him quite ill and covered with a nasty looking rash. Unfortunately, the circle of illness continued as the medications changed. Finally, through much "trial and error research," we were able to identify the culprit medication, and he began to improve, but the progress was very slow.

To make matters worse, Dick's twenty year-old cat, Chin, began dying at the same time as Dick was recovering from surgery. She had kidney failure and was not making it to her cat box. I had two severe cases on my hands and thought to myself at the time, "Why do women spend so much time in life taking care of the bottom half of bodies, humans and otherwise?"

Dick's post surgical troubles served to remind me of how important it is to check everything from medications to other bothersome requirements, such as making sure an enema is given before surgery. The fact that Dick did not have an enema prior to the surgery resulted in an episode the next day that caused him excruciating pain for more than an hour.

I think it is also vital to be present at the hospital during a patient's stay to help facilitate their recovery. Nowadays with the problem of understaffing in some hospitals, it is prudent to stay in the room with the patient at least until he is comfortable and mobile. Recently, a friend of ours took a nasty fall in his hospital room. Disoriented from his pain medicine, he was not clear about his whereabouts when he awakened. He headed for the restroom not realizing he was hooked up to an IV and fell on the way. After inadvertently tearing out the needles, he called for help but no one heard him and he was not able to come to his feet. He remained on the floor for a long time. Having someone else in the room helps prevent such scenarios and patients can go home in one piece.

Dick was happy to be home even if he had suffered his setback. After six weeks, Dr. Fishman gave him permission to practice operating his new implant. He was thrilled with his amazing apparatus and the ease with which it could be operated. Now all he needed was the right wife. Since I was the going candidate, I became the Mrs. Because of the timing of the surgery and his marriage proposal, I was never sure if it was love or research that precipitated our union.

I must admit that I was a bit overwhelmed by his enthusiasm for his new technological wonder. That is not to say that I was not enjoying our intimacy, but I wanted Dick to understand that as a menopausal female, my hormone level was not the same as when I was twenty. And, frankly, Dick had such a new lease on life that I could not keep up with this man who was acting like the Titan of Testosterone.

### Talking About the Sexual Solutions

When Dick began to openly discuss his operation with others, he gave me what we refer to in the South as the "vapors," which is a cross between anxiety and embarrassment. I was fine as long as our communication about sexual subjects was confined to the two of us. Once another person was added to the conversation, however, I became uncomfortable. I don't mean that Dick brought up the subject in the course of a dinner table conversation, but if men asked him about his surgery, he did forthrightly answer all of their questions.

Although I was not so willing to publicize this part of our lives, Dick remained true to his mission. He had the "Somebody's gotta do it, because it's important" attitude. My perspective in regard to openly discussing sexual matters was "Somebody *else* has gotta do it." Eventually, he won, even though it never occurred to him that, perhaps, I should have been part of the decision to open our personal life to the public. As I stated before, how could I, as Dick's wife, act as if I didn't play an integral part of this new adventure, especially when noted medical journalists were gathering and publishing intimate facts about Dick's case? Once when Dick was the keynote speaker at a large meeting focused on impotence at the National Institutes of Health, he had everyone laughing when he told the attendees, a large group of journalists, that he didn't know how he had become the "Impotence Poster Boy."

After a fairly definitive article about Dick's situation appeared in the *Reader's Digest*, I became apprehensive about public reactions, particularly the public that happened to know us personally. Fortunately, no one made an issue of it except to compliment Dick on his willingness to help other men by being frank about his own problems and his struggle to overcome them. I assumed they wanted to know more about our situation, but most of them refrained from asking because of the subject matter.

Although I still am not completely comfortable with such discussions, I felt better about my hesitancy when I read a number of articles convincing me that I am in good company. It appears that many physicians typically find it difficult to discuss sexual topics with their prostate cancer patients or other patients for that matter, particularly if the wife or partner is present. The majority of medical schools offer at least one course on human sexuality, but these courses are generally not required, so many physicians do not learn how to facilitate a conversation that might reveal a sexual problem.

To complicate matters, men rarely volunteer such information or communicate their problems for months or even years after they experience some degree of impotency. It is important to openly discuss these issues with the physician. Time is lost and medical solutions are delayed if a conspiracy of silence develops between the prostate cancer patients and their physicians about sexual subjects.

Since a urologist is accustomed to such discussions, a woman can help by encouraging her partner to visit his urologist and openly discuss every facet of his problem, especially since it could be related to other causes like vascular obstruction or specific medications and not necessarily wholly associated with prostate cancer treatment. By being open with the urologist, he can more easily determine if there is an available solution or a better treatment for the man's impotency

Women should also never underestimate the significance that most men place on having an erection and being able to perform sexually. To illustrate the importance of a continuing sex life, a doctor friend of ours told us about an eighty-year-old patient of his, who had a severe heart condition and had to use an oxygen tank to breathe properly. When the man entered our doctor friend's office wheeling his oxygen tank, the doctor immediately inquired about the nature of his visit.

119

He was surprised when the gentleman asked for a Viagra prescription. The doctor quickly told the man that he absolutely would not give him the Viagra prescription, because of the man's general poor health and heart problems. Disappointed that the doctor would not prescribe the potency pills, the patient headed out the door exclaiming to the doctor and the nurses who were in hearing distance that he would keep looking until he could find someone who would heed his request.

Another eighty-year-old man told his doctor he wanted to lower his sex drive. Amazed, the doctor said he was surprised at the man's request since most men wanted to raise their sex drive. The older gentlemen winked and said he wanted his sex drive lowered from his head down to you know where. Those two stories were perfect reminders to me of the importance of sex in a man's life at any age and under any circumstance.

Both men and women are curious about the penile implant and the sexual satisfaction it provides. Women have asked me, "Does the implant really feel the same?" It does not feel exactly the same. By that I mean there are subtle differences but nothing major. American Medical Systems, the manufacturer of the "gold standard" penile implant has indicated that there can be minor changes in the length and girth of the penis but this does not necessarily happen. One must realize too that differences occur as a man ages, regardless of extenuating problems like prostate cancer treatment. I also recognize that nothing is the same as I mature, including my personality, hair, body and general health. Life is great if you learn to accept and adjust to the changes! In other words, hair dye is a good solution to my now gray hair. The implant device is a good solution for sexual difficulties.

The next questions I often hear are, "Does the implant feel natural and does it look natural?" That one is a definite and easy "Yes!" Men and women are afraid that the implant will not look natural but it is very natural looking. One such question came from a man.

Recently, Dick received a phone call from a prostate cancer survivor. I explained that Dick was not home, so the man asked me if I would mind answering a question about the implant. I gulped but assured him that I would be happy to be of help. He explained that he and his fiancé had talked about his getting an implant, but they were not really sure what a "real live recipient" thought of it. I answered his questions, including the one about its natural appearance, as succinctly as I could and tried to put aside my apprehension about discussing this sensitive subject. I could tell that he was embarrassed to be questioning me but put aside his feelings as well in order find out what he needed to know.

Then there is the question, "Is 'it' strange, because 'it' is not spontaneous?" The device takes very minimal time for the man to operate, so spontaneity is not sacrificed. Furthermore, with the advent of drive-by shootings, security alarms and other startling events, I am not sure I want surprises anymore. I may not be old enough to be thinking in terms of having a heart attack any time soon, but nowadays a big surprise might precipitate one.

Because of our own experiences, Dick and I have since learned a great deal about the reactions of others to the sexual aspects of prostate cancer. In our opinion, the couple's basic relationship, including their ability to communicate openly, is the most important factor in their ability to deal with the sexual issues. I have continued to insist that Dick and I maintain open communication about the side effects of my diabetes and porphyria as well as his prostate cancer. Whereas, Dick openly discusses prostate cancer facts and figures with the general public, he is less likely to communicate with me on an intimate level. From what I have observed over the years, men communicate in a less empathetic manner than women, probably as a means for them to maintain their sense of control and competency or give others the appearance that they are capable individuals.

At first, I was concerned that Dick would mistake my conversations about "touchy" subjects as unhappiness with him. I was afraid that he would feel hurt or rejected by my comments or questions. Many women can identify with my concern as they spend their lives putting the feelings of others above their own. But continuing this process of walking the fine line of my needing to converse about our situation and his wanting to avoid the subject was not emotionally healthy for me. Therefore, I changed my course of inaction and insisted on more openness from Dick. He still has a tendency to answer my questions and comments quickly and not fully, but he is working on changing this life-long diversionary habit of avoiding difficult subjects or conflict. Reminding him in subtle ways about the importance of "talking through" our dilemmas has helped us find a better plane of communication on sexual matters.

Some men who are so uncomfortable talking about their sexual troubles with their wives or partners that they will only share their problems with their doctor or male friends, if at all. This can be so very distressing. When a man does not use his wife or partner as a major link in his support system, he generally raises her level of frustration and, in turn, increases the possibility that she will raise her own barrier in the relationship. My insistence on "real" communication has, I think, prevented future conflict in our marriage in light of our health problems. Communication is the essence of intimacy, and women seek and respond to intimacy.

I have read that men's and women's ratings of their marital satisfaction can be predicted by adding up how often they have sex and subtracting the number of times they have arguments. In response to this advice, Dick and I try to maintain a peaceful time together filled with much laughter. In case we do ever have a serious conflict, good advice is nearby: We have a pillow in the guest bedroom that has a funny Phyllis Diller quote, *"Don't go to bed angry. Stay up and fight!"*

Another gripping point is that some men have mentioned their fear of losing their wives because of their cancer and/or subsequent sexual problems. Studies indicate that the reverse is true when their basic relationship is good. According to the American Cancer Society, no increase of divorce is noted among cancer patients and most people have observed that cancer and its side effects have strengthened their commitment to one another. This is not to say that some women have not left their partner when they discovered that he had prostate cancer and became impotent to some degree after treatment. I have rarely heard of this happening, although I do know two men who have been dealt this painful blow. In my naiveté, I was stunned when I found out that the women actually left for this reason.

On one occasion, I took it upon myself to call one of the gentlemen in question. I know him very well, so I was not hesitant to assure him that he was a remarkable man and that his level of potency had nothing to do with his stature in life or his manhood. I was so hurt for him, but I knew that my conciliatory words were not the answer. I decided to write him a letter about the impression others had of him, his intellect, his goodness, his integrity and all the things that really matter in life. I asked Dick to speak with him to reiterate my concerns and plaudits as well as talk to him about his sexual future and share all of the different options Dick had undertaken to achieve a solution to his own sexually related problems. Their talk was encouraging and boosted the man's ego considerably. Plus, Dick was able to encourage him to take charge of his sexual problem and deal with it. Our friend had the penile implant surgery and is quite satisfied with it as is his wife. Happily, the couple has reunited, and they are striving to improve their emotional and physical relationship.

The other friend, whose wife left because of his potency problem, has found a new sweetheart with whom he is very compatible and recently reported that he is happier than ever.

These are good endings to potentially disheartening stories but telling such stories doesn't always help when someone is experiencing heartache. So as a woman, if you come across one of these hurt men, you can help by sharing these or similar accounts as well as a bit of your comforting nature with them. A woman's tenderness and understanding goes a long way in this busy, sometimes uncaring world. An invitation to join you and your husband for dinner always helps, too. My friends kid me about my lousy cooking, but believe me, when people are lonely or hurt, they don't care about the food; they care about the company.

Communication is important in another light. I have had women tell me that sometimes they don't want to try to have sex until their partner at least talks to them about seeking a better solution to his erectile dysfunction. Otherwise, the experience can be either too frustrating or too disappointing. Rather than experience disappointment, some women merely withdraw and show little or no enthusiasm for lovemaking. I have heard a number of these objections and comments about the strain it puts on the relationship when the two cannot work on the problem together.

A man and woman must recognize the difficulties in their sexual life and be willing to create an atmosphere that is conducive for honest communication. In my view, ignoring problems, sexual or otherwise, will only compound them. Important in this process is a man's willingness to not react in anger, hurt or in any intimidating way. Most women by nature pull back from confrontational issues. When this happens, honest communication goes by the wayside and is often difficult, if not impossible to regain.

Interestingly, some men feel so desperate about their sexual problems, and their feelings of inadequacy are so overwhelming, that they encourage women to leave them or push them so hard they eventually leave. Strange as it sounds, I have been told this by several wives of prostate cancer survivors. Being pushed away is extremely depressing and frustrating for the women who love these men and want to help their partner find a renewed life after prostate cancer. Perhaps, these men are testing the commitment of the woman they love, or they may feel alone in their plight and inadequate as a husband and lover.

In her book, *Sexuality and Cancer*, Dr. Leslie Shover discusses the psychosexual changes surrounding cancer treatment: what to expect physically and emotionally, how to communicate with loved ones, which feelings are specific to gender, the effect of feeling unattractive, the fear of divorce, depression and numerous other sexually related issues.

In one study she cites, almost 70% of prostate cancer survivors have varying degrees of erectile dysfunction (ED) problems. In fact, approximately 140 million men worldwide suffer from some measure of ED. These figures demonstrate that men are certainly not alone in their sexual plight and the fact that most of them have a woman standing beside them should demonstrate the female level of commitment.

That is why it is so important for all of us to communicate about our difficulties and the solutions we have found to overcome them. Communication is always a major part of the answer to most every problem. With this in mind, Dick set out on his own awareness campaign.

### *Filling the Information Void*

Despite his own Goliaths, Dick is concerned about other men who have been diagnosed with prostate cancer. For ten years, he has spent 30 hours a week in this field and continues to spend that amount of time learning about the disease and all of the exciting new developments and then educating other men on the subject. Dick is a highly educated scholar who holds a number of degrees, including several masters and a Ph.D., and is endowed with a propensity to learn more than a person needs to know about a subject, in this case prostate cancer. In short, Dick flunked retirement and has taken on a new volunteer career as a prostate cancer advocate.

His first venture into sharing his knowledge took place two weeks after his surgery. Because of the information void that existed at that time, he headed for the Baylor Medical Library and delved into the journals and medical texts on prostate cancer. After he felt sufficiently educated on the subject, he sent 600 letters to his friends and business associates centering on what he had learned about prostate cancer and encouraging them to take a PSA test. Not only did he receive an overwhelming response to this letter, but he also learned that there were a number of men who were diagnosed with prostate cancer as a direct result of his urging.

After six more months of studying and spending additional time in the library, he sent an even more comprehensive letter to 1200 men and had the same positive response. This time he began receiving 1-2 phone calls each day from men who had been newly diagnosed with prostate cancer. Dick took the time many doctors did not have to answer all of their questions with in-depth explanations of the treatment options.

Most men also wanted to talk about the "unspeakable" side effects of prostate cancer treatment: incontinence and impotence. Because of Dick's unassuming nature, his vast knowledge about prostate cancer and his willingness to openly share his own trials with these two side effects, men gravitated to him to discuss their unique physical and emotional problems. To date, he has counseled more than 3000 men one-on-one, in one to two hour sessions. This is like spending eight hours a day, forty hours a week for two and a half years at the office on the telephone.

As his knowledge increased to the expert level, it became evident that he had much to offer the world of prostate cancer. So several years after his first letters, he was asked to submit a paper to the *Journal of Urology*, which is the leading peer-reviewed scientific journal in this field. It is my understanding that his was the only paper ever written by a layman published in this prestigious journal at that time. This paper opened many doors for him, including participation on fifteen of the most important national committees and invitations to present papers at technical meetings attended by the leading doctors and researchers in this field.

During this period, he developed a simple technique for comparing the research dollars being spent per death on prostate cancer, breast cancer and AIDS. The differences were startling with prostate cancer on the low end of the funding totem pole. These numbers have been quoted four times on The Larry King Show and referred to by the President of the United States once. More importantly, they have also been used with the Congress to help to increase research funding for prostate cancer from 30 million dollars in 1991 to over 400 million dollars in 2001.

Dick has also spoken with many women, some of whom pressured their men into taking a PSA. In a number of cases, as mentioned earlier, women were the ones who would research the treatment options, particularly when their husbands were in a state of denial. It was endearing to me to hear them as it precipitated memories of the days I struggled to learn about cancer treatments for my deceased husband, James. Near the end of his life, I heard about a new treatment for pancreatic cancer that was being studied in Japan. Desperate for help, I tracked down the President of the Japanese company in his limousine in Paris, which is quite a feat for a housewife in Texas.

At first, he sounded extremely irritated, "How were you able to convince my office to give you my personal number?" "Sir," I replied, "I love my husband and love is the greatest motivator in the world."

Then I began to quickly tell him our plight always interjecting how much I loved and cherished my husband. When I finished my explanation, he thanked me for calling him and offered to help me any way possible. I will never forget his kindness even though James died before we were able to wade through the red tape to secure the treatment. So it is with many other women. They absolutely will not stop searching until they find a remedy or some form of help for the man they love.

## *The Scare*

A year before Dick and I married, he had his first PSA scare. About a week after he had his semi-annual PSA test, the results of which had always been less than 0.1, he realized he had not received the results. He called the urologist's office but was unable to reach the urologist or his nurse. The clerk who answered the phone volunteered to look it up in his file. She said, "It is really low, 0.3!" Because the number had moved upward from less than 0.1 to less than 0.3, it most likely meant that Dick was undergoing a treatment failure and that the cancer had returned. Very concerned, he told the clerk that if the nurse did not call him in two hours, he was coming to the office. It was a tense wait.

When the nurse returned his call, Dick asked her two important questions. First, he wanted her to check if the doctor had changed laboratories and if so, he wanted to know the minimum PSA that the new lab reported. She explained that they did, in fact, change laboratories and the minimum at the new lab was less than 0.3. The clerk's seemingly minor mistake of missing the "less than" sign on the report gave us a major scare.

Dick firmly reminded the nurse to tell the doctor that he should not have changed labs, and if the change was necessary, he should have advised all of his patients of the change in advance. He then wrote a five-page letter to the urologist telling him how such mistakes, like the one he experienced, could have tremendous impact on patients and their families. Dick also began informing prostate cancer survivors of the importance of remaining with the same laboratory for their tests if possible. If a lab change was made, they should not rely on a test result that came up "tilt" until it was verified.

Not long after Dick and I married, he had a second PSA scare. During a consultation with Dr. Fishman, who was not his primary urologist, Dick mentioned that it was time for his PSA and asked if he could have his regular PSA at Dr. Fishman's office rather than making another trip to his regular urologist. Dr. Fishman agreed and sent Dick's blood sample to the laboratory his office used. Without thinking, Dick had violated his own rule about changing laboratories.

We then left for our lake home near San Antonio. The three-hour drive was fairly anxious, because PSA tests are always reminders that cancer can return unexpectedly. Outwardly, Dick did not seem to be concerned, but having lived the cancer scenario, I knew he was apprehensive and would remain so until he heard that the PSA result was still less than 0.1. I tried to assure him that all would be well without appearing alarmed myself. Several days later, Dr. Fishman called and said he had bad news. The test came out 0.3. Dick asked him if the result was 0.3 or less than 0.3 and what was the laboratory minimum. Dr. Fishman explained that the result was 0.3 and the minimum was 0.1. It was a gloomy report but to lighten his spirit, Dr Fishman suggested that Dick take the test again in thirty days.

Dick steeled himself for the ensuing battle with advanced prostate cancer. I was not willing to take the PSA report at face value, so I insisted that there could be an explainable discrepancy and that he return to his primary urologist and redo the test at the original laboratory.

We headed home, and I called my daughter, Lelia, followed by a call to my friends, Joanne Davis and Sandra di Portanova, to ask them to undertake a prayer vigil for Dick. Joanne and Sandra and I had made it a point to pray together almost every day for many years, so it was second nature to bring our joys and troubles to one another and then to place them together in our Creator's hands.

Prayer is both comforting and exciting to me as I have seen astonishing results from effectual prayer. Since I am a guilt prone person, prayer also helps me forgive myself for my failures and inabilities. I can easily identify with the following supplication and wish I could find out who wrote it. Since it was sent to me many times over email, I gather there are numerous others who share the sentiment:

## A Prayer for Every Day

*So far today, God, I've done all right. I haven't lost my temper, haven't been greedy, nasty or self-centered. I am really proud of myself. But in a few minutes, God, I am going to get out of bed, and then I'm going to really need some help.*

Interestingly, I have since read data from a study conducted at the University of California, San Francisco, indicating that people who were prayed for fared much better than the group who received no prayers. To add more import to this study, those who fared better did not even know the people who were praying for them or that the study was transpiring. The wonderful thing about faith is that it isn't dependent upon test results or studies. It is an indescribable knowledge that our lives are in God's control, the best place we could ever be. So keep this in mind, stick with the same laboratory if it is a good one and stick with God, who is the same yesterday, today and forever.

We maintained our prayers as we awaited the results of the follow-up PSA. Sandra was in Acapulco and Joanne and I were in Houston, but distance didn't stop our threesome. We joined together in daily telephone conference calls with Dick's situation as the focus of each prayerful call. I called Lelia independently, because I wanted to savor every conversation with her. Lelia is a special woman, who genuinely loves her new stepfather and was diligent in her prayers for him.

Dick did not alarm his sons with the latest report. They had already lost their mother, and he didn't want to concern them about his future health. Dick's sons are wonderful men, who love and respect their father and again would have given him an extra measure of support during that trying time.

Hallelujah! The first thing I did when we received the news that Dick's PSA retest was less than 0.1 was to phone Lelia, Joanne and Sandra so that we could thank God together. Dick rationalized that changing laboratories was one answer but rightly discerned that the main answer was in the form of a Divine blessing.

The next test the following year at his regular laboratory was less than 0.1 as well. With this new lease on life, we set out together in high gear with a firmer commitment to join other prostate cancer survivors and their families to change the world of cancer, like the story of the mighty river formed one drop at a time.

# 7.

## The Beginning—Basic Information about the Prostate

**I** started my journey of inquiry for this book by asking what I thought every man and woman would like to know: "What is the prostate, and where is it located in the body?"

The prostate gland is a little understood part of the male reproductive system. It is a small chestnut shaped organ deeply embedded in the body sitting at the base of the bladder at the floor of the pelvic cavity. It is situated in front of the rectum, below the bladder,

The prostate itself surrounds a portion of urethra below the bladder. The urethra is the tube that runs from the bladder out through the penis. Interestingly, a French surgeon Ambroise Pare coined the word *prostate* from the Greek word meaning "stand before" because of the prostate's proximity and its relationship to the bladder. The prostate is surrounded by major arteries, veins and many very delicate nerves. Both urine and sperm pass through the prostate before they leave the body.

Normally, the prostate does not affect urine flow. However, as a man ages, the prostate begins to enlarge. It can become so enlarged that it constricts the urethra causing varying degrees of blockage to the flow of urine from the bladder. This condition, **Benign Prostatic Hyperplasia** (BPH) can be treated easily.

The major function of the prostate is to produce a clear, mildly acidic fluid consisting of proteins and other chemicals that nourish sperm and are important for male fertility. This prostatic fluid, called semen, helps transport the sperm formed in the testicles, contains chemicals that help sustain the sperm after it has left the penis. This fluid also protects the reproductive and urinary tract if it has an invasion of bacteria that have entered the body through the urethra.

As an aside, men can remain fertile or able to produce sperm and father children well into their seventies. Fertile men with prostate cancer, who want to father children, need to collect and bank their sperm for later use before they have treatments. Prostate cancer treatment may not necessarily affect a man's fertility or his potency, but it is quite probable. Although men can remain fertile without a prostate or seminal vesicles, they cannot remain fertile with both removed. A radical prostatectomy is, in effect, like having a super vasectomy. Because most men who are diagnosed with prostate cancer are over fifty, they are not as concerned about fertility issues as younger men.

Another fascinating fact is that all male mammals have some type of prostate, but only men and dogs contract prostate cancer spontaneously. Women do not have a prostate but do have a similar pelvic structure, the Skenes gland, which has no obvious purpose.

The prostate is pea-sized when a man is an infant. During a man's aging process, the prostate grows into a walnut sized gland as it is exposed to the male hormone testosterone. If these hormones are removed, the prostate gland will not fully develop or can shrink. As the size and weight of the prostate slowly increases so does the level of the PSA, which is why a rapidly rising PSA in a younger man carries such significance. Since there are already a number of variables, including variables in laboratory techniques, it is important to continue testing at the same laboratory. This way the test results are consistent and not confusing as they were in Dick's case when he changed labs for the sake of convenience and when his urologist changed labs without telling him.

The prostate is covered by a thin capsule, usually weighs about twenty to thirty grams and measures about an inch and a half wide at the widest point at the base, which is at the top just beneath the bladder. A muscular valve that controls urine flow, the inner urethral sphincter, is at the top of the prostate and base of the bladder. The function of this smooth muscle valve is to close involuntarily at the instant of ejaculation to prevent semen from going into the bladder. The external urethral sphincter, sometimes called the striated sphincter, is the muscle used to voluntarily control the urine flow. It is located just below the prostate. The prostate has two sides or lobes, left and right, separated by the urethra. It is also divided into zones; the peripheral zone, which can be felt during a DRE and is the zone where most of the prostate cancer occurs, the anterior zone, which covers the largest area, and the transition and central zones which lie close to the urethra.

The prostate accounts for only 0.03% of the body's weight yet it is the most troublesome gland in the body. It is composed of two distinct types of tissue: **connective (stromal) and epithelial (glandular) tissue**.

The connective tissue is a fibrous structure, which supports mini glands within the prostate and supports the epithelial tissue. PSA is produced in the epithelial tissue and is secreted when the fibrous connective tissue contracts and expands. One simple explanation of the process is that it is like a complex "sponge" with five zones. The crevices in the "sponge" fill with prostatic fluid being made by the epithelial cells lining the crevices. Most of the glands in the prostate are located near the rectum in the peripheral zone, where most cancer develops. The transition zone surrounds the urethra and is where most of the BPH arises. (BPH is not a precursor to prostate cancer.)

It is important to note that most cancer arises in the epithelial cells and are **adenocarcinomas or glandlike carcinomas.** A transformation of these epithelial cells, called **prostatic intra-epethelial neoplasia** (PIN), is believed to be the earliest manifestation of prostate cancer, but its importance is still not totally understood.

PIN begins to appear when men are in their 20's, and when they are in their 50's, almost 50% of them have PIN. It is not cancer and, therefore, does not require treatment, but is believed to be a precursor to cancer. Pre-cancerous changes in the size and shape of the cells can be seen in the biopsy specimens under the microscope. PIN cells, which are not seen outside of the capsule of the prostate, can coexist with prostate cancer. They do not appear to metastasize and can exist without ever becoming prostate cancer. However, PIN can have either a low or high grade. If the grade is high, the likelihood of developing cancer is increased, so monitoring that condition is important.

Prostate cancer behaves differently than most cancers because the natural history or rate of change of a tumor, which is generally low, is nonetheless unpredictable. However, as described above, prostate cancers having higher Gleason grades double in volume much faster than those with lower Gleason grades. Usually, cancer cells start growing slowly and then replicate at an increasing speed and in an unpredictable manner, particularly after they reach bone. In prostate cancer, the growth of the tumor may follow this pattern, or it can remain slow all of a man's life. Interestingly, some large tumors may be indolent while the smaller ones may be very aggressive. Aggressive and slow growing cells can coexist in the same tumor.

There can also be a great difference between **clinical** and **pathological prostate cancer**. Clinical prostate cancer is what the clinician can detect outwardly via PSA, scans, bone pain, etc. Pathological prostate cancer is what the pathologist determines after examining biopsy tissue microscopically. If a tissue sample is examined microscopically and is found to have cancerous cells, it does not mean that that tumor would ever be a problem even if left untreated. On the other hand, it could cause a very severe problem.

Autopsy provides another dramatic example of the pathology of these tumors in men who died of causes unrelated to prostate cancer. Of these men who had a postmortem examination by a pathologist, a few who were in their twenties, had latent cancer cells. The percentage of men having latent cells increases as the age of the man increases. At age 80 about 80% of men have prostate cancer cells, but most of these cells are latent. The lifetime risk of being diagnosed with clinical prostate cancer is 15%. Apparently, prostate cancer can exist in the prostate for many years without becoming aggressive. In fact, only a small number appear to be aggressive. This is another example of the need for a way to determine which cells may be clinically significant in the future.

# 8.
## More Useful Procedures

*Bone Scans, Computed Tomography, Prostascint and Magnetic Resonance Imaging*

**S**ometimes metastasis is suspected following initial diagnosis or is discovered in the lymph nodes during a radical prostatectomy. If metastasis is suspected or has already occurred, tests are in order to determine the extent and location of the metastases. In these circumstances, a bone scan is generally performed.

### The Bone Scan

The bone scan does not detect cancer *per se*, but rather it detects damage in the bone structure from certain bacterial infections, fractures, arthritis or cancer. If, however, a man has been diagnosed with prostate cancer and the bone scan indicates extensive damage, the cause is usually cancerous bone involvement. This damage is generally seen in the hips, thighs, spine, and pelvis.

To perform a bone scan, the patient is injected with a specially designed radioactive tracer. The tracer circulates through the bloodstream, and filters into the bones. A gamma scan can then detect areas where more of the tracer has accumulated, which may indicate cancer.

### The CT Scan

If a man is initially considered to be a high-risk patient, which means that his PSA and/or Gleason Score are high, or if he has experienced a surgery failure and the PSA is rising, his doctor might order a CT Scan to determine if one or more of the lymph nodes are enlarged. This would be indicative of cancer and would, therefore, mean the patient may not be a candidate for surgery or radiation.

Computed tomography, which is also called a CT Scan or Cat Scan, takes pictures of the interior of a patient's body to locate cancer. To locate prostate cancer a patient is generally injected with a specific dye to enhance the image. He is then placed flat on a table with his midsection ringed by the scanner. An x-ray beam rotates around his midsection and takes a series of interior pictures from a number of different angles. A computer then transforms these pictures into cross-section images that display varying densities of the tissue. The radiologist then determines if the densities indicate cancer either in the prostate or in areas surrounding the prostate like the lymph nodes, bladder, etc.

The CT scan is used primarily to find a sizable mass, which is unusual in early stage prostate cancer. It is not helpful at indicating small cancers outside of the prostate.

Although CT scans are expensive, the CT equipment is shorter and larger in diameter than the MRI "tunnel" and thus, does not cause claustrophobia. Again, it is important to seek expertise in this field in order to acquire the most effective scan.

## ProstaScint

ProstaScint is a relatively new imaging technique. Monoclonal antibodies are used to deliver radioisotopes to the tumor via the bloodstream. The antibody attaches itself to the cancer. A gamma-ray camera is then used to detect the location of the radioisotopes. This test can sometimes indicate if there is node involvement, which is helpful to determine if localized therapy, such as surgery or radiation therapy, would be beneficial. Generally, ProstaScint is used when there is a recurrence of prostate cancer after localized treatment or in patients who are at high-risk for non-organ confined prostate cancer at diagnosis.

## The MRI

Magnetic Resonance Imaging (MRI) reveals an astonishing internal image of the prostate but is only rarely used. Although the images from an MRI are amazing, the MRI is costly and the images cannot be used to accurately stage prostate cancer. However, an endo-rectal coil is now improving the images.

During an MRI scan, the machine generates a magnetic field that induces electrical charges in the patient's body. A sensor picks up the charges and a computer transforms these charges into pictures of the interior portion of the body being examined. These pictures are generally clearer and more detailed than those of a CT scan. However, an MRI is more expensive and more difficult for some patients than the CT scan.

The patient lies as motionless as possible on a stretcher like surface. He is then rolled into a large tube, which is open at both ends and serves as a circular electromagnet. Although the procedure is painless, many people are overly anxious when a loud clanging noise begins during the MRI, and others find the chamber so confining that they suffer claustrophobia. The length of the procedure, forty-five minutes to an hour, is also a negative factor. Some individuals even need tranquilizers in order to continue the test. A relatively new development is the open MRI machine, which is much less distressing to claustrophobics.

On the other hand, when I had an MRI, I found it to be less invasive and easier than other procedures. I also appreciated the fact that I was not subject to radiation of any kind. When I had an MRI recently, I remained still and prone in the chamber and constructed my list of errands and structured my next writing project.

A friend of ours is Dr. Raymond Damadian, the inventor of the MRI. At present, he is perfecting an MRI room and MRI operating room. To me, this is the best of all testing worlds, because you are in room where the MRI results are projected on a screen. The surgeon, who is also in the room, views the cancer and removes it at the same time. This allows the surgeon to see if he has removed the entire tumor and less visible cancerous cells. The implications of this type of MRI are more far reaching than I can fathom.

## Chest X-Ray

The physician might suggest having a chest x-ray to make sure that prostate cancer has not spread to the lungs, but it is not done routinely. Prostate cancer does not usually spread to the lungs in the early stages, although it can in the late stages of the disease.

# 9.

## Exciting New Developments

Prostate cancer research is exploding with new discoveries, including four exciting new developments described below:

### Vaccines

We are presently hearing a great deal about vaccines for prostate cancer. These are not vaccines in the traditional sense, whereby they would immunize a patient against acquiring prostate cancer. These vaccines are formulated for a specific patient and injected. The B-cells produce antibodies and the T-cells attack the cancer. This is easy to say but hard to do; however, scientists are making good progress.

### Monoclonal antibodies

Monoclonal antibodies work in a somewhat similar way. These antibodies are injected in the bloodstream and are programmed to attach themselves to just the prostate cancer cells. In other words, they have the ZIP code of these cancer cells, and antibodies go to the intended Zip code. When they arrive at their destination, they can be used to deliver chemotherapy or radiation therapy directly to the cancer cells. This has worked very well in mice and is now in Phase I trials in men. There are already nine FDA-approved monoclonal antibody drugs and more than 70 in trials, half of which are for cancer. This is extremely important research and might well be one of the silver bullets we have been seeking for so long.

### Gene therapy

Gene therapy has become a huge field, due in part to the recent completion of the Human Genome Project. There is feverish activity aimed at discovering which genes are either over-expressed or under-expressed in, for example, prostate cancer. Once they determine which genes are which, they will try to eradicate the bad ones and replace the good ones that are missing. This technology has the potential of eventually producing cures for specific types of cancers.

### *Anti-angiogenesis*

Anti-angiogenesis is another exciting area of cancer research. We have known for a long time that cancer cells need additional blood supplies to grow and that they are capable of performing manipulations on their own to secure these new supplies. This is known as angiogenesis. If we can prevent this from occurring, the cells cannot spread and might even die. Once again, it works in mice but not very well in men—yet.

# 10.

## If Prostate Cancer Spreads

Prostate cancer sometimes spreads to the lymph nodes near the prostate, as well as to bones and other organs. It spreads to the bone in 80% of late stage patients. When this occurs, men can be pain free but most often suffer moderate to severe pain in the spine, ribs, pelvis and skull. It is not uncommon in this situation for a man to have multiple bone fractures. Also, if the tumor is located on the vertebrae, spinal cord compression and nerve damage can occur.

If the prostate cancer has metastasized to the bone, the treatment varies depending upon whether the patient has had prior treatment. For example, if bone metastases develop in spite of the initial hormonal therapy, further hormonal treatment is given with drugs that **suppress androgens**, like **Nizoral** (ketoconozole). These drugs have not been very beneficial.

**Chemotheraputic agents** are also being given to reduce the cancer as well as the pain. Drugs called **biphosphonates** are being studied for prostate cancer. These drugs, including **Aredia**, help prevent bones from breaking. External beam radiation is also used to reduce bone pain in about 80% of patients, but it can only be used until patients reach their lifetime dose limit. If so, or if there are multiple bone metastases, **intravenous radioactive drugs** like **strontium-89** (Metastron) and **samarium-153** can be used. If needed, these drugs can be repeated.

Healthy eating habits, vitamins and exercise can strengthen bones, while smoking and heavy alcohol intake can cause bone loss. However, if a man is on testosterone or has bone loss or bone metastases, he needs to check with his physician before embarking on an exercise routine.

## *If Surgery or Radiation Fails*

If the PSA starts to rise after surgery, there are three options to consider: **adjuvant radiation, hormonal therapy** or **no immediate treatment**.

First, it is important to determine the location of the cancer, which is causing the PSA to rise. If it is located in the vicinity of the prostate, adjuvant radiation therapy might be tried. When a man has had a radical prostatectomy and he has positive margins or positive seminal vesicles, often a decision is made to follow the surgery with adjuvant radiotherapy. The results appear better if the treatment is given early.

If there is lymph node involvement or metastasis to the bone, hormonal therapy is indicated. When it should be initiated is the next question. Some physicians recommend that it be started immediately, and others recommend that the patient wait to begin the therapy. When to begin hormonal therapy to achieve the maximum benefit is not clear.

If radiation was performed as the primary treatment and the PSA begins to rise again, it is rare that a "salvage" prostatectomy is performed. The irradiated tissue is ordinarily too damaged for surgical removal without creating unacceptable additional side effects. Also, the morbidity that accompanies this procedure is considered excessive.

# 11.

## What About Pain?

One of the great problems with advanced prostate cancer is pain. Because prostate cancer spreads to the bone and spine, it can be extremely painful. What complicates the problem is that men often suffer in silence or refuse to take sufficient medication to overcome intense pain for fear of addiction. Many men also have difficulty expressing the intensity of their pain, because they don't want to be labeled as "complainers." Another problem is that some men delay taking painkillers until they can no longer bear the pain, thinking that if they take pain medication early on in the pain cycle, the drug will lose its effect. This is an unfortunate misconception, because the medication dosage can be adjusted to the level of pain or changed to a more powerful drug. As for the fear that the use of pain medications leads to addiction, it is generally held that taking pain medications for real pain rarely leads to addiction. And for those who are concerned about cost, pain medications are generally very inexpensive.

To add to the pain problem, some physicians, who are inexperienced with cancer pain, do not prescribe enough painkiller. Perhaps, they are not aware of the amount of medication needed to make a cancer patient comfortable. Perhaps, they fear that their patient will become addicted or fear that the patient will become overmedicated and die from an overdose. Whatever the reason, you can and should demand appropriate pain management if the pain remains a problem.

I had an unfortunate experience in this regard. Not long before James died, two relatives were milling around in the bathroom cabinet looking for aspirin. They noticed the array of pain medications lined up on a special shelf in the same cabinet. One of the women criticized me for having so much medicine and commented that James was probably addicted to pain pills. Her remarks hit me like a land mine.

I explained that James had varying degrees of pain and he had a number of different conditions, so he needed a number of various medicines for each condition. For example, after his surgery for pancreatic cancer, he had intense pain from his muscles being cut in his abdomen and needed strong pain medications. When he developed pleurisy, he needed an anti-inflammatory. I continued with my examples to illustrate why we had various kinds of medicines and asked her to note that most of the bottles were still full. My initial explanation didn't phase her. She continued her insinuations even after my showing her that the majority of medications were not painkillers.

I proceeded to explain that James' doctors at M.D. Anderson Cancer Center had prescribed all of the medicines he was receiving and that I met with them frequently about each drug and its effects. They assured me that he was not taking an excessive amount of medication. Furthermore, I told her that MDACC had a special pain management department and that I had attended programs at the pain clinic and consulted with the pain specialist on a number of occasions, who also assured me that James' medication levels were good. Mostly, I thought, "Why don't these women think more about the suffering James is enduring than the pills he is taking to relieve it?"

Their hurtful remarks so disturbed me that I called James' doctor and talked to him about the incident. He was very comforting and told me I was a great caretaker and wonderful wife and should not be disturbed by the comments of these women. He also added two things that gave me some delight. "Where are they when you give him his 2AM medication and when he needs a 4AM warm compress, and by the way, which medical school did they attend?" That helped my wounded spirit.

I share this story with you, because many people will have ideas that may conflict with your own or your physician's.

When you are working hard to help your partner, it is difficult to deflect some of this negativity. As with most ideas, consider the source. Next, when you know and love a person intimately, you develop instincts about that person that others, including the doctors, do not have. Don't be afraid to make your instincts known to the doctor. Good doctors are very willing to listen to a person's "feelings" about their own illness or the illness of those they love.

Attending educational sessions at the pain management clinic at MDACC gave me knowledge that has helped me with the many sick people who are placed in my path. The most important fact I learned was to stay ahead of pain. In the past, I thought a person should only take pain medication when the pain became intense. In fact, people use less medication in the long run when they start the medication as the pain begins. This prevents pain from getting out of control. When pain is under control, people can return to their normal daily lives, so the sooner they can achieve pain relief the better.

Pain is also responsible for reducing appetite and the ability to keep active while it increases depression. Depression, in turn, adds to the loss of appetite and a person's desire to keep physically and mentally active. Thus, the cycle of pain continues. This is an area in which a man's partner can help considerably by insisting on proper pain management, including insisting on having the doctor prescribe enough medication, if necessary, to keep her partner comfortable. With the many excellent pain medications, in various strengths, that are available today, there is no excuse for anyone to endure undue suffering.

The essential issue is to make sure the patient has pain relief. However, because opiates like morphine slow the bowels, doctors suggest that it is good to drink plenty of fluids and, perhaps, even take a stool softener to avoid constipation, which can add to the pain problem.

Pain precipitated by advanced cancer can sometimes be treated with **radiation** targeted to painful areas and with **strontium-89 (Metastron)**, a radioisotope that is injected and acts on new sites of metastasis. Although some men experience an increase in pain the first week after treatment, the strontium-89 passes the healthy bone and is quickly absorbed by the metastases in the bone. Relief generally occurs within a few weeks. The radiation dose is quite low and half of the radiation leaves the body within hours of the injection. The other half of the strontium 89 remains in the body for 50 days and makes a significant impact on the pain. When the initial injection is no longer effective, further injections may be given until the bone marrow begins to be affected. Because the injection is radioactive, the doctor will provide the patient with a means to carefully collect the urine as opposed to disposing of it in the toilet.

Spinal cord compression can occur with advanced prostate cancer and is very painful. It is caused by cancer invading the bones and must be treated immediately and aggressively to prevent the risk of paralysis. Since it is extremely important to treat spinal cord compression early, call the doctor at once if you note any of the following symptoms: severe back pain along with numbness in the toes, difficulty walking, leg weakness, urinary retention or constipation.

When this condition is suspected, the patient first will be given an MRI to image the spine and determine if there is indeed spinal cord compression. If the compression is evident, he will be given corticosteroids for forty-eight hours. Depending on the evidence at reevaluation, the patient may receive targeted radiation to the compression area or an operation to ease the pressure on the spinal cord.

You might also ask your physician how to prevent broken bones, which can be another serious problem with advanced prostate cancer. When cancer invades the bones, they become

148

brittle and break easily but don't heal easily. These breaks are known as pathological fractures. Basic steps to protect the bones are extremely beneficial, like not walking on rough or uneven terrain, removing any furniture or obstacles in the house that might cause someone to stumble or fall. These and other simple measures can prevent painful broken bones. Sometimes, doctors put pins in the weight bearing bones to prevent such breakage. This seems to work well when the cancer covers a large area of the bone.

If the pain or obstruction gets so severe that it robs a man of his appetite, there are appetite-stimulating medications available or very nutritional liquid supplements, like Ensure. Ensure and its counterpart, Sustacal, are readily available at local drug stores. Visiting a nutritionist may also prove very helpful. If these measures fail, your doctor can insert a gastromy tube, through which liquid food can pass to the stomach to help provide much needed nutrition.

Many patients also take advantage of the beneficial effects of complimentary pain management techniques like yoga, biofeedback, acupuncture, massage therapy and above all prayer. And doesn't the Good Book tell us that a cheerful heart is good medicine?

# 12.

## Complementary Medicine

Complementary medicine is another name for alternative medicine. I think the former is a much better name, because in most instances, this approach complements traditional medicine and is not just an alternative.

Bill, a friend of ours, has implemented what he calls integrated medicine because he integrated complementary and traditional medicines. When Bill was diagnosed with prostate cancer, he had a PSA of 39, a Gleason grade of 8 and was incurable at diagnosis.

He first had an orchiectomy, surgical removal of the testes, and began a combination of other therapies. He and his wife adopted a strict vegetarian/macrobiotic diet, which was extremely low in fat and included no animal fat. He set aside a quiet time for prayer, mediation, and mind/body exercises like tai chi. In addition, he has scheduled acupuncture treatments to boost his immune system.

After his orchiectomy and these additional therapies, Bill's PSA remained undetectable for four years. When his PSA began to rise, he was given radiation treatments and continued his previous therapies. His PSA quickly returned to its undetectable state. Although some people may contend that this last six years of remission is due solely to the radiation treatments, Bill feels that it is the result of integration of both the traditional radiation treatments and the complimentary therapies.

Michael Milken, the financier and philanthropist, is another proponent of a strictly low fat diet to prevent cancer and to hold back the growth of his own advanced cancer. His commitment to this belief has resulted in two excellent cookbooks filled with very low fat, healthy recipes, *The Taste For Living Cookbook* and *The Taste for Living World Cookbook*.

He is also committed to regular exercise and stress reduction. As a result of combined hormonal therapy and his significant lifestyle change, his cancer remains under control after almost ten years.

Dr. William Fair was the Chairman of Urology at the Memorial Sloan-Kettering Cancer Center, one of the premier cancer hospitals in the world, from 1984 until 1997. As one of the country's preeminent prostate cancer surgeons, he did not embrace complementary medical therapies until he was diagnosed with colon cancer. In 1994 he began feeling poorly but chose to ignore his state of health despite his wife's nudgings to seek help. Finally, she convinced him to go visit his doctor, who diagnosed him with colon cancer. Unfortunately, when the tumor was removed, it had already spread, so he was given chemotherapy.

After the conventional chemotherapy failed, he wanted to seek other routes to defeat the disease. He began to investigate other approaches outside the realm of traditional medicine and decided to try complementary therapies including dietary changes, yoga, meditation and herbal preparations. He and a group of researchers also began to develop a vaccine using his own cancer cells to be used when the existing therapies are no longer effective.

Next, he learned about SPES, a combination of eight Chinese herbs from the same company that produces PC-SPES for prostate cancer. He contacted Dr. Sophie Chen at the Brander Cancer Research Institute in New York, who had been working on the SPES for many years, and she sent him the compound. He implanted some of his own cancerous cells into nude mice in his laboratory. After the mice grew the cancerous tumors, he fed them the herbs, and the tumor shrank. Most noteworthy was that the mice did not die from the cancer.

With this kind of result in mind, Dr. Fair began taking SPES along with adopting a new low fat diet and other complementary therapies, and the tumor shrank. He also attributes his improved health to his own personal transformation. Because of his own benefit from complementary treatment, he and his son started HAELTH, a complementary health center, and he became the associate editor of the journal, *Alternative Therapies in Health and Medicine.*

Another area in which Dr. Fair hoped to have an impact was to help physicians understand the role of complementary medicine and the need for an integrative approach to include complementary medicine. Most doctors are beginning to appreciate this theory and apply it to their practices, particularly since so very many diseases are associated with a person's lifestyle.

One of the experiences that dramatically influenced his thinking was when he attended a program where he learned about the significance of focusing on expanding life rather than extending life. Dr Fair also began concentrating on the distinction between being cured and being healed. I never understood this distinction until a cancer patient, who was staying with us while being treated at MDACC, shared her experience with me. "I saw the doctor today, and he told me the cancer is widespread now and that there is no other medical treatment available for me. I am bothered by that thought, but I also have this inexplicable feeling that I am healed in the greater sense of the word. I can't explain it, but it is a real feeling." She had reached an understanding and spiritual plane that I did not share. Some people never reach the state of being where they enjoy every moment they have left on earth, regardless of whether it is a long or short time.

In addition, Dr Fair wrote a powerful article wherein he discusses not only the effect of some complementary treatments but also the power of words on our emotions and health. In the medical realm, a doctor can crush a patient's hopes entirely with a few insensitive words and conversely give the patient hope with a few encouraging words.

In the article, he also suggests that a doctor not make statements indicating how long a patient might live as it may have some immeasurable mind effect.

I understand this entirely. Because of my own experience with porphyria, I have a propensity to notice my unusual metallic pallor when I am not well. Normally, I maintain a very positive outlook about my condition and healthy future. If an unfamiliar doctor appears overly concerned when he notices my pallor or asks about my symptoms, I suddenly become overanxious. Conversely, when the doctor who diagnosed me, Dr. George Penton, would enter my intensive care room and announce that I looked great and would be going home soon, I would immediately improve. As proof of this effect, my blood tests usually showed marked improvement after his visit.

In the past, it has been difficult to acquire information about complementary medicines, but complementary medicine has become so important that the National Institutes of Health have established The National Center for Complementary and Alternative Medicine (NCCAM). This center was born out of the groundswell of patient interest. It is dedicated to exploring complementary/alternative healing practices in the context of rigorous science, as well as training complementary and alternative medicine researchers and disseminating authoritative information. Another significant improvement is that the National Cancer Institute now has a Division of Cancer Prevention.

# 13.

## Attitude

I have been so impressed with the attitude of many patients, but one man, Anthony Herrera, immediately comes to mind. Anthony, a good friend of ours, has been a star on the long-running soap opera, *As the World Turns*. In January 1997, he joined the community of cancer survivors when he was diagnosed with mantle cell lymphoma, a far more aggressive and deadly cancer than prostate cancer. Since that time, he has become the first person with that disease to receive what is called a "mini" stem cell transplant. But there was nothing "mini" about it. During his four-year struggle, he suffered severe infections, indescribable pain, seizures and a stroke. Amazing as his case is, he is now back at work playing the proverbial bad guy, John Stenbeck, on *As the World Turns* and is in the midst of writing *The Cancer War*, a book about his miraculous victory.

The doctors and nursing staff at MDACC, who performed the transplant, deserve great admiration for their brilliance, compassion and very hard work. But Anthony deserves immense credit, too. Despite the dreary outlook for his future, Anthony pressed on against all odds with the courage of John Paul Jones, the tenacity of Alexander the Great and the demanding nature of Leona Helmsley. He focused on those things which would get him through the horrible ordeal that lay ahead of him, including seeking psychological support, laying aside distractions, concentrating on his healing, not wasting his time on fruitless efforts, accepting love from those of us who loved him, openly expressing his anxieties and fears and visualizing himself well again. All of these things were not easy for Anthony, especially when he was a long way away from his apartment, friends and job in New York City.

Another friend whose attitude we admire is David Smith. David had advanced prostate cancer. Before he quit work and long after he was no longer able to bear the load of a full time job, David dedicated his life to others. He exemplified the Word, "It is better to give than to receive." He volunteered at the hospital, helped at prostate screening programs, attended support group meetings and shared in the administrative responsibilities of these groups. His generosity of spirit was endless as if he was attached to a never-ending supply of joy. David attributed his positive attitude to the gratification and happiness he felt when he was involved in a project to help other people. He had a wonderful purpose and because of it, he had a very long remission.

There is a familiar scripture found in the book of Isaiah that can transform our attitudes:
*But those who wait upon the Lord will renew their strength. They will mount up with wings as the eagles. They will run and not grow weary. They will walk and not faint.*
Those words have kept me and many other men and women intact when we were about to fall apart under the pressure of a serious illness. The promise that He will renew us is a very powerful incentive to trust that our lives will improve. Knowing that alone is enough to change one's attitude. But how do we "mount up with eagle wings" and recover that sense of control over our lives?
My way is to pray, trust in the promise in Isaiah, spend time with my family and sit quietly at my computer and write my thoughts. Being with my dearest friends is also valuable for me. I mention dearest friends, because I have found that being with acquaintances with whom I lack emotional intimacy just doesn't do the trick in tough times.

Dick's coping mechanisms are to pray, be with his family and sit at his desk with a pile of papers two feet high, the higher the better. Our good friend, Tom Redmond, who is a prostate cancer survivor, tells me that his spirit lifts when he rides his horse or feeds the buffalo on his ranch in Colorado. Every person has his or her attitude adjustment technique.

# 14.

## Your New World Is Not Easy,
## But He's Got The Whole World In His Hands

Facing cancer and worrying about the future are not easy. Both the men who are diagnosed with prostate cancer and the women who walk the journey with them often have many difficult days, but facing them together with their lives in the right Hands lightens the burden. One distinct advantage to finding yourselves in such an abyss is that you can very quickly find clarity in your lives, particularly in what is important in life and what is not. You learn quickly that there are powers to help you that are much greater than the abyss: the love of God, the love of family and the love of friends.

A friend of mine illustrated this point to me when I was in horrible grief over the loss of James. We were sitting around a campfire one night under the kind of Texas sky that it so big its enormity added to my loneliness. We watched the fire quietly for a while when he pushed one small log from the center of it. Slowly the log began to diminish in intensity until it lost its flame, then its light, then its heat and then it died. He said, "So life goes when you separate yourself from other people and from your Maker." When I saw the burnt log lying beside the roaring fire, I knew that log was like me. God was not finished with me yet, but I was too overcome and too embarrassed about my "neediness" to seek help to carry on in life and too grieved to walk in His purposes. I learned a lot that night from a simple log and a friend who cared enough to encourage me to join the world again.

Here are a few propositions that may help during the prostate cancer journey:

*Loss of control over our lives:* The diagnosis of prostate cancer can make a man feel powerless over his life and bleak about his future. It is difficult to deal with every day activities when you have been so severely and quickly cut to the bone. If a woman can bear some of his personal everyday responsibilities, she can usually watch the metamorphosis of a man overwhelmed by his circumstances into one who has regained control over his life. And remember to turn to the One who has got the whole world in His Hands.

*Guilt:* Sometimes a man blames himself for causing his family to be burdened with a financial and emotional burden because of his condition. Unwarranted as these feelings are, they are real to him. The woman may also feel guilty over her inability to change his diagnosis or improve the course of his disease no matter how wonderfully she takes care of him. Many women have told me that they overcame their own feelings of guilt by concentrating on giving their spouse loving support. Support groups and counseling can be very helpful in this situation. And remember to turn to the One who has got the whole world in His Hands.

*Exhaustion:* Exhaustion can have profound effects for both the patient and the caregiver. In fact, the symptoms can be the same: forgetfulness, inability to concentrate normally, emotional swings, decreased sexual interest, irritability, etc. Exhaustion can make you feel defeated and can open the door for more illness to tramp into your body. The world tells us to fight, fight, fight but most often we need to rest, rest, rest! Rest is healing. And remember to turn to the One who has got the whole world in His Hands.

*Depression:* One common feeling faced by most prostate cancer patients and their families is depression. Receiving the news of a prostate cancer diagnosis is hard to digest emotionally. It can even lead to clinical depression, which manifests itself in symptoms, such as changes in sleeping and eating patterns, shutting out friends, withdrawing from normal enjoyable activities, and outwardly exhibiting emotional changes. Many patients and their spouses don't seek help, because they think that feeling severely depressed is a normal part of dealing with prostate cancer and there is no help. If you or your partner has symptoms of depression, you might ask your doctor for a referral to a good counselor to you help cope with the emotional impact of the diagnosis and treatment of his disease. And remember to turn to the One who has got the whole world in His Hands.

*Anger:* Ongoing anger can be destructive. Since I was born with a sense of humor, I am never one to hold anger long. Somewhere along the way, I find something humorous in almost every situation. Laughter makes it hard to cling to anger for a long period of time. I do know that many men and women have expressed anger over their diagnosis of prostate cancer. Again, support groups and professional counseling may help rid them of such a stressful and potentially destructive emotion. And remember to turn to the One who has got the whole world in His Hands.

*Loneliness:* When you are walking in what feels like a vast wilderness, it always helps to know that you are not alone. The number of men diagnosed with prostate cancer is now over a million men in the U.S., and almost all of them have a strong woman by their side. Hold on to each other and to the many hands and hearts of family and friends and even strangers reaching out to you. And remember to turn to the One who has got the whole world in His Hands.

# 15.

## Statistics

Expanding your spiritual life, boosting your immune system, improving your general overall health and expanding your loving relationships are all important in changing the following statistics.

Statistics

The American Cancer Society has published the following "Key Statistics About Prostate Cancer" on their website:

- About 200,000 men were diagnosed with prostate cancer in 2001;
- Ninety-three percent of all men diagnosed with prostate cancer survive at least 5 years, and 72% survive at least 10 years. These figures include all stages of prostate cancer;
- At least 70% of all prostate cancers are found while they are still *localized* (confined to the prostate). The 5-year relative survival rate for men with localized prostate cancer is nearly 100%;
- Twelve percent of prostate cancers have already spread to tissues near the prostate when they are first diagnosed. The 5-year relative survival rate for men whose prostate cancer has spread regionally is about 94%;
- Of the 9% of men whose prostate cancers have already spread to distant parts of the body at the time of diagnosis, 33% will survive at least 5 years.

The American Cancer Society also estimates that 31,500 men in the United States died of prostate cancer during 2001. This translates into the sad truth that one man will be diagnosed with prostate cancer every 3 minutes and one will die every 17 minutes. One of these 31,500 men could be our husband, son, son-in-law, partner, nephew or good friend.

### What Can We Do To Change These Statistics?

*Never doubt that a small group of committed citizens can change the world. Indeed, it is the only thing that can.* --Margaret Mead

As women, we can be powerful instruments to change these statistics. We need only look at the colossal difference made over recent years in breast cancer awareness and in private and public funding of breast cancer prevention, detection and research programs.

There are many extraordinary organizations already in place that are making great strides for prostate cancer. You can unite with these groups and participate with their abundance of fundraising events. Most cities have Fun Runs, Baseball games, Father's Day dinners and any number of activities dedicated to raising money for prostate cancer. Your involvement can make the event successful. Knowing that your participation in such activities will help fund the research that can change the life and health of the man you love is also gratifying to the soul.

As you may recall, some women, like Florence Baskas, start a project of their own. To raise money and heighten awareness about a disease that had a family predisposition like prostate cancer, Carla Rehnquist used her daily walking routine as the focal activity of her fundraising campaign. She started by planning a very scenic 100-mile trek. Then she set about collecting donations for every mile she walked. Next, since the disease had been diagnosed in several men in her family, she solicited family members to participate as drivers to follow her or walk with her.

They placed a large magnetic sign describing their mission on their truck and set off into the countryside. The photos they sent me showed a happy family enjoying a wonderful adventure, stopping to sightsee, picnic and camp along the route.

Their brightly colored sign that hung on the side of the van and the sight of a family of "walkers" drew a great deal of attention. In fact, local and national media picked up the story, so their research fund-raising campaign turned into a forceful public awareness blitz as well. I have always thought this adventure or something similar would be a good event for a family reunion project if prostate cancer runs in the family.

Prostate screening programs always need volunteers to man the registration tables and other various administrative tasks. Most local hospitals have existing screening programs and have specific weeks or days that the screening takes place. They always need assistance during those busy times.

Betty Gallo, lost her husband, Congressman Dean Gallo of New Jersey, to prostate cancer at the age of 58. She has been instrumental in lobbying his former colleagues in Congress for more research funding for the disease and in establishing The Dean and Betty Gallo Prostate Cancer Center so that other men, and the families who love them, can live longer, healthier lives. Betty asserts that her goal is to advocate the importance of early detection, awareness, and education about prostate cancer and to play a part in reducing the suffering that often accompanies the disease.

Whatever you choose to do to help improve the prostate cancer statistics, you will be gratified at the end of the day. I have chosen to write a book and give speeches on prostate cancer as well as open our house to out-of-towners in need of a home during their treatment at M.D. Anderson Cancer Center or Baylor College of Medicine. All of these endeavors have given me great satisfaction and have in some small way contributed to "making cancer history."

# 16.

## The Last Word

Before this book was completed, I was speaking with the publisher about why I would need another week to finish it. I reached over my sofa and lovingly showed her a photo of my daughter, Lelia, and my granddaughter, Elizabeth Grace. "These two paid me an unexpected visit last week," I said, "and if I have not learned through this journey in the cancer world that being with them is more important than anything I have to do or say or write, then nothing I share it the book is worth reading."

So it is with each of you. Your healing partnership goes beyond the education, research and treatment that you and your beloved experience together. It also goes beyond your partner's physical healing from prostate cancer. It is not merely the absence of disease. Your healing partnership is an opportunity for both of you to transform your lives and your relationship and to intensify the beautiful intimacy and love affair that you already share.

God bless you in your journey.

# For Your Information

## Organizations

**American Cancer Society**
1599 Clifton Rd., NE
Atlanta, GA 30329
404-320-3333; 800-ACS-2345
www.cancer.org

**American Dietetic Association**
800-366-1655
www.eatright.org

**American Foundation for Urologic Disease**
1128 N. Charles Street
Baltimore, MD 21201-5559
410-242-2383;800-828-7866
www.afud.org

**Canadian Cancer Society**
10 Alcorn Avenue, Suite 200
Toronto, Ontario M4V 3B1
Canada
416-961-7223; 888-939-3333

**Cancer Care, Inc.**
1080 Avenue of the Americas
New York, New York 10036
212-302-2400; 800-813-HOPE

**CaPCURE** (The Association for the Cure of Cancer of the Prostate)
1250 4$^{th}$ Street
Santa Monica, CA 90401
310-458-2873; 800-757-CURE; 310-458-8074 fax
E-mail: capcure@capcure.org ; www.capcure.org

**Harvard Center for Cancer Prevention**
665 Huntington Avenue
Building 2, Room 105
Boston, MA 02115
617-432-0038; 617-432-1722 fax

**HAELTH**
212-334-9600; 877-4HAELTH
E-mail: info@haelth.com; www.haelth.com

**Impotence World Association**
800-669-1603
Email: info@impotenceworld.org; www.impotenceworld.org

**Men's Health Network**
202-543-6461; 888-MEN-2-MEN; 202-543-MHN1
www.menshealthnetwork.org

**The National Cancer Institute Information Services**
Building 31, Room 10A31
31 Center Drive, MSC 2580
Bethesda, MD  20892-2580; 310-435-3848; 800-4-CANCER

**The National Center for Complementary and Alternative Medicine (NCCAM)**
NCCAM Clearinghouse
P.O. Box 8218
Silver Spring, Maryland 20907-8218;
888-644-6226

**National Association for Continence**
P.O. Box 8306
Spartanburg, SC 29305-8310
800-252-3337
www.nafc.org

**National Prostate Cancer Coalition**
1156 15th Street, NW
Washington, DC 20005
202-463-9455
www.4npcc.org

**Two Against One:  Couples Battling Prostate Cancer**
877-550-9624

**US TOO International, Inc.**
930 North York Road, Suite 50
Hinsdale, IL 60521-2993
630-323-1002; 800-808-7866
www.ustoo.com

**Visiting Nurse Association of America (VNAA)**
800-426-2457; 888-866-8773; 617-523-4042;
617-227-4843 fax
Email: vnaa@vnaa.org;
www.vnaa.org

# Cancer Centers

**The Brady Urological Institute**
The Johns Hopkins Hospital
Baltimore, Maryland 21287-2101
410-955-6707
www.prostate.urol.jhu.edu

**Center for Prostate Disease Research (CPDR)**
Department of Surgery
Uniformed Services University of the Health Sciences
240-453-8900; 202-782-8105; 240-453-8912 fax
www.cpdr.org

**M.D. Anderson Cancer Center**
1515 Holcombe Blvd.
Houston, Texas 77030
713-792-6161; 800-392-1611
www.mdanderson.org

# U.S. Government Information

**Cancer Information Service (CIS)**
800-4-CANCER;301-402-5874 fax
A free service of the national cancer institute -- A national information
and education network, CIS is your source for the latest, most accurate
cancer information for patients, their families, the general public, and
health professionals. CIS responds to calls in English and Spanish.

**Cancer Liaison Program**
Food and Drug Administration
FDA Room 9-49CFH-12
5600 Fishers Lane
Rockville, MD 20857; 301-827-4462 Email: OSHI@oc.fda.gov

**Cancer Clinical Trials Listing**
www.fda.gov/oashi/cancer/trials.html
An alphabetical listing of cancer organizations with extensive
information about cancer treatments and clinical trials.

**CancerNet™**
http://cancernet.nci.nih.gov
Provides links to cancer information including portions of the PDQ
database, information about ongoing clinical trials, NCI fact sheets,
publications, CancerNet™ News and CANCERLIT® abstracts and
citations.

### Cancer Prevention and Control, CDC
http://www.cdc.gov/cancer/
Focuses its cancer prevention and control resources in five priority areas, including the Prostate Cancer Control Initiative.

### Healthfinder™
www.healthfinder.gov
Provides information on selected online publications, clearinghouses, databases, websites, support, and self-help groups, government agencies, and nonprofit organizations.

### MEDLINEplus
www.nlm.nih.gov/medlineplus/
Designed to direct you to resources containing information that will help you research your health questions.

### National Network of Libraries of Medicine
800-338-7657
Directs health professionals, educators, and the general public to health care information resources.

### PubMed
http://ncbi.nlm.nih.gov/PubMed/
Internet information retrieval service that provides free access to MEDLINE®

### CancerTrials
http://cancertrials.nci.nih.gov
The National Cancer Institute's Resource for Cancer Clinical Trials Information.

### PDQ®
http://cancernet.nci.nih.gov/pdq.htm
NCI's Comprehensive Cancer Database, contains peer-reviewed summaries on treatment, screening, prevention, and supportive care; a registry of approximately 1,500 open and 9,500 closed clinical trials from around the world, and directories of physicians, genetic counselors, and organizations that provide cancer care, including FDA-approved mammography screening facilities.

## Manufacturers of Erectile Dysfunction Products

### American Medical Systems
Penile/Sphincter Implants
10700 Bren Road West
Minnetonka, MN  55343
800-328-3881 www.visitams.com

**Pfizer, Inc.**
Viagra oral medication
35 East 42$^{nd}$. Street
New York, New York 10007
888-4-VIAGRA
www.viagra.com

**Pharmacia-Upjohn**
Caverject penile injection
95 Corporate Avenue
Bridgewater, NJ 08807
800-253-8600
www.impotent.com

**Timm Medical Technologies**
Vacuum devices
6585 City West Parkway
Eden Prarie, MN 55344
800-438-8592; 612-947-9410; 612-947-9411 fax
Email: customerservice@timmmedical.com

**VIVUS, Inc.**
MUSE urethral suppository
605 E. Fairchild Dr.
Mountain View, CA 94043
888-367-6873
www.vivus.com

## Prostate Cancer Videos

**"Not by Myself" Talking About Prostate Cancer.**
877-550-9624 for a free video
Billy Davis Jr. and His wife Marilyn McCoo, plus other patients and their families share inspiring personal experiences.

**"Take Charge: For Men Newly Diagnosed With Prostate Cancer"**
Produced by: State of the Art, Inc. 888-275-2605

## Great Reading

**Dr. Patrick Walsh's Guide to Surviving Prostate Cancer; also, The Prostate: A Guide for Men and the Women Who Love Them**
Dr. Patrick C. Walsh and Janet Farrar Worthington

**Prostate & Cancer: A Family Consultation**
Dr. Phillip Kantoff

**The Lovin' Ain't Over: The Couple's Guide to Better Sex After Prostate Disease**
Ralph and Barbara Alterowitz

**My Prostate and Me: Dealing With Prostate Cancer**
William Martin, Ph.D.

**Power For Living**
Jamie Buckingham

**Prostate Cancer, revised edition**
The American Cancer Society

**Prostate & Cancer: A Family Guide to Diagnosis, Treatment & Survival**
Dr. Sheldon Marks and Dr. Judd Moul

**Sexuality and Fertility After Cancer**
Leslie Schover, Ph.D.

**The Taste for Living Cookbook: Mike Milken's Favorite Recipes for Fighting Cancer**
Beth Ginsburg and Michael Milken

**The Taste for Living WORLD Cookbook: More of Mike Milken's Favorite Recipes for Fighting Cancer and Heart Disease**
Beth Ginsberg and Michael Milken

**Eating Your Way to Better Health: The Prostate Forum Nutrition Guide**
Dr. Charles E. (Snuffy) Myers, Jr., Sara Sgarlat Steck, RT, and Rose Sgarlat Myers, PT, PhD

**Anatomy of An Illness**
Norman Cousins

**Viagra: A Guide to the Phenomenal Potency-Promoting Drug**
Dr. Susan Vaughn

**The Bible**
God

# A Note about the Publisher

Winedale Publishing is a small press founded in 1996 that specializes in creative non-fiction, including medical memoir, and literary fiction.

We are a member of the Texas A&M University Press Consortium, a group of university presses and independent publishers located in Texas. Other members of the consortium include Texas A&M University Press, Southern Methodist University Press, Texas Christian University Press, University of North Texas Press, Baylor University Press, Texas Review Press, McWhiney Foundation Press, the Texas Historical Society, and the Dallas Morning News.

Our books are available in any bookstore, directly from our website, www.winedalebooks.com, from the consortium website, www.tamu.edu/upress; or call toll-free to order: 1-800-826-8911.

## Also from Winedale Publishing

---

### HOME SPUN and SUPPER TIME
### by Leon Hale

The warm and gently funny style of Leon Hale is the perfect tonic for hard times.

> "Reading these short meditations is like settling in with a box of bourbon candy: It's hard to stop with just a few, and if the booze doesn't buzz you, the sugar will. His enthusiasm for life…is undeniably infectious."—*Kirkus Reviews*

*Home Spun*  Journalism/humor/0-9657468-2-8
*Supper Time*  Non-fiction/memoir/0-9657468-3-6


### AFTER GREAT PAIN: A New Life Emerges
### by Diane Cole

A *New York Times* Notable Book and one of *USA Today*'s top books of the year, *After Great Pain* remains both timely and of great use to readers traumatized by disaster or grief. Diane Cole's method is to couple the findings of professional researchers and clinicians with the story of her own heartbreaking personal experience—coping with a multitude of family illnesses and the after effects of being held hostage by Muslim extremists.

> "Cole's book is by turns harrowing…consoling and finally inspiriting."

*--Washington Post Book World*

Memoir/Psychology/0-9701525-5-8
*New in Paperback*

## DRINKING WITH THE COOK
### by Laura Furman

In this critically acclaimed short story collection, Laura Furman reminds us of the literary pleasures to be derived from close examination of seemingly uneventful lives. Possessed by "a passion for the safe and permanent," her characters react to the impossibility of fulfillment in complex and unpredictable ways.

"Her luxuriant histories...are sure and exact, drawing the
reader in and rarely loosening their grip."
--*New York Times Book Review*

"*Drinking with the Cook*, by Laura Furman, wonderfully
captures the creepy dislocation of people who are on the
verge of being abandoned by those they think love them."
--*Detroit Free Press*

Fiction/Literature/0-9701525-2-3

## RÍO GANGES
### by David Theis

This striking first novel depicts in vivid, visual terms the confusion and pain that a father's desertion can create throughout a young man's life. Complex and moving, it reminds the reader of love's redemptive power and the ways children can require us to live.

"This powerful novel takes you through a rugged emotional and
physical terrain and makes you experience it—feel it through your
pores."—*Phillip Lopate*

"*Rio Ganges*...is passionately, elegantly wrought—a forge in which the
materials of erotic obsession, parental devotion and the beauty and
poverty of the Mexican landscape are merged and purified."
—*Emily Fox Gordon*

Fiction/Literature /0-9701525-6-6